The Tools for Building a More Superior You

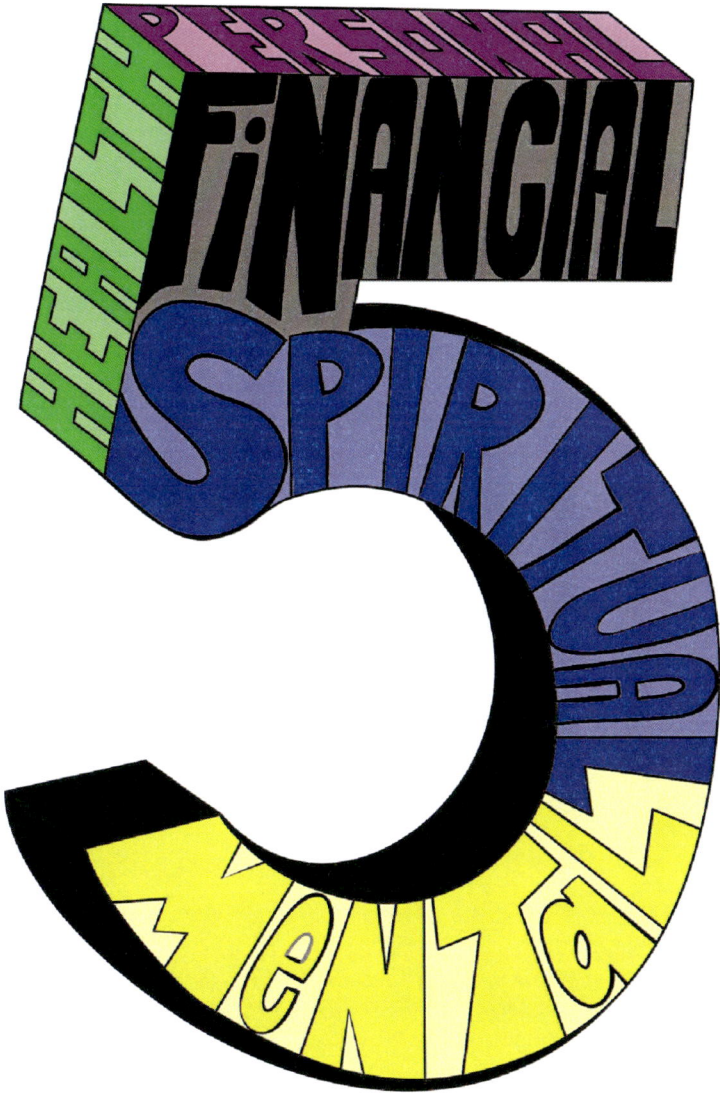

Image by Nicolas Delgado

First paperback edition November 2019

D.O.P.E. Publishing

ISBN: 978-1-943586-43-1

Treat Me Like I'm Famous!

Love Me Like I'm Dead!

Table of Contents

Thank You

To my family and friends no longer here in the physical, to the people who have been by my side over the years and most importantly to the gang, I love you!

To my grandma, thank you for teaching me love, discipline, loyalty, perseverance, and diligence at all times.

To my mother, thank you for instilling in me that I should always speak my mind, and that, as long as I am alive, there is nothing on God's green earth I cannot overcome because as you once told me, "When there is life, there is hope."

To my neighborhood, thank you. The lessons I have been through have taught me to stay rational and to never worry about facing a predicament I can't handle because I have been through it all.

To my pops, thanks for having sex with my mom. I love you, my nigga!

Finally, to my second-grade teacher, Mrs. Pandolfe, thank you, and to my college advisor, Ms. Givens—I wouldn't have graduated college without you. I appreciate every one of those 45 minute meetings that went past 45 minutes and the endless emails you replied to anytime I had an issue.

Glossary - Bag Talk

Baglike - to do something that will contribute to being a better you

Bagly - to do something conducive to your superiority

Unbaglike - to commit an act detrimental to the elevation of yourself

Unbagly - to do something against your superiority

Splashisms - the theory of tools being utilized in regard to self-elevation advanced by Maurice Eastwood

'Off the strength' - due to the fact; the explanation of your actions

- This book also contains shared experiences that will broaden your outlook on various situations presented, based on the valuable life lessons and tools that aided in building a more superior me.

As you begin the process of unlocking a more superior you, I would like you to stop and take note of the opening page for each of the 5 bags. There will be a page with an ombre gradient scale for each color that represents one of the 5 bags. For example, the color that represents the Spiritual Bag is blue. Self-reflect and identify your current place at this moment in life when looking at the gradient pages. The closer you are to the subtleness of the color represents how much negative energy and recessive light you are allowing into your bag (you). Unless internal changes are made, you will continue to be pulled away from the depth-of-self and further removed from your substance. You should drown in the depth of each color, so deeply that no light is entering your bag. Remember, the light is what you do not want; it is the baggage and its association to negative traits and energy. The subtleness of each color consists of things such as negative thoughts, friendships that are no longer needed, ignoring signs, not loving yourself, etc. Keep in mind, you don't want to see light; this is not a tunnel or one of the metaphors where you have to see the light. This is a bag, and when you look at any bag, the light is at the top. You want to drown, as I mentioned earlier, because you have substance—only light things with no substance (hollow) float at the top.

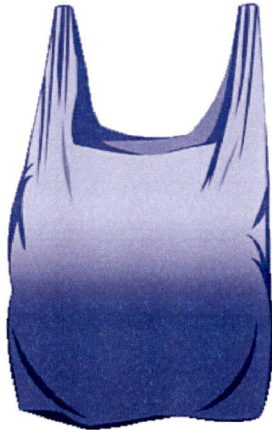

Image by Shavoy Banks

"Spend all that time trying to be people, meanwhile they all want to be you." – Maurice Eastwood

<u>Foreword</u>
By - G - $TAK aka (Yuk)

The essence of a man's influence is directly related to his evolution, growth, and emotional maturation. This book will give you a front row seat to truly understanding the perspective by which (Splash) sees his process of shifting and aligning his paradigm to that of impact, uplifting ideas, and personal development. As you read and examine *The 5 Bags*, you will explore within your own self areas-that need recalibrating and possibly a complete manufacturer's reset. This book allows the ability for one to honestly look within themselves and make a true assessment of where you put your energy and where the fulcrum has shifted, thus disrupting the balance.

I have had the distinct pleasure of observing Maurice (Splash) develop himself from a brash young man in high school to a philanthropist, business owner, mentor, coach, motivator, and person of humble transparency. I have seen him, over many years, contribute to his community by way of massive Thanks-giving dinners, feeding over 500 people. He organized AllXity basketball tournaments to raise money for scholarships, book bag and school supply giveaways, celebrations allowing individ-uals to adorn themselves in their finest garments, created pop-up shops to support local artists, planned and executed holiday coat and clothing drives, and supported local businesses and entrepreneurs. All of this was done after he observed a need in the community that he embraced and took action to affect a positive impact.

Maurice is constantly encouraging and challenging people to read at least one chapter of a book or fifteen minutes a day to increase vocabulary, knowledge, and perspective on any topic. He is most certainly effusive in his pursuit of a higher self through understanding and accepting how emotional baggage can affect your outlook on life, thus embracing it to unravel the spiritual knots to let the energy flow.

There are many who say they do it for the culture or that *they stay ten toes down* in the community, but not many carry the same pedigree in selfless sacrifice as Maurice (Splash).
If you want true correlation to his walk and the bags he breaks down with precision, look no further than his everyday actions. Every New Year, his challenge is for people to save money by saving the five-dollar bills you possess daily and banking one dollar bills and change at the end of the day. He is a huge advocate for mental health reconditioning through therapy, and he is transparent about the need for it, especially in a traumatized community.

This book will require you to take notes, read and reread multiple times, stop and pontificate on certain sections for a deeper personal understanding, have dialogue with others to expound on particular interpretations, and look within to allow for evolution, growth, and emotional maturation.

"Cause haters wanna shoot everything that shines."
– Russell Tyrone Jones

Preface

Around 6:22pm on Sunday, August 27, 2017, just two hours after my annual AllXity School Supply Giveaway, somebody pulled up on the side of my car at the stop light and sent shots into my car—in broad daylight, for a reason I am still unaware of to this day.

Niggas is trash though; I ain't get hit. Simply because it wasn't my time, and it wasn't meant for the God to go out like that. It also means those prayers my loved ones say when they talk to God on my behalf were heard. The situation was and still is weird as fuck. I sensed that shit coming. I felt like I had an outer body experience. Weird as fuck, right? I know. I was tired as hell driving home, so I wound the window down to let the breeze keep me awake. A car pulled up in the left lane, not all the way parallel to me. Something told me look over my shoulder, whatever that voice was. Thank you! I looked and saw a person with just a black hoodie tied so tightly, I couldn't even see their face. I looked straight ahead and thought to myself, "Why the fuck is there a person with a hoodie on in the hot ass sun?" I looked at them again about five seconds later and was looking directly into the barrel of the gun. Several shots went off, but I managed to get out of the passenger side of the jeep fast as hell without getting hit. (God's doing, not mine). I still don't even remember how I got out of the car; I'm just glad I wasn't wearing my fucking seat belt.

This was the second time niggas tried to take my life and failed. That type of shit puts you in a cold ass space. It's a naked feeling. It was so real, I thought it was fake; I thought I was dreaming of getting shot. It was the fastest yet slowest five to ten seconds of my life. Every time I blinked for about a year, I could see that shit replaying. Endless cold sweat filled nights. I damn near didn't stop at a red light for a year. I'm not sure what's worse: not knowing who did it or the fact that I'm possibly dapping up a person who could be the shooter.

But anyway, to the shooter: "Fuck you, you bozo. You had one goal, and you failed. That's all you ever do in life is fail, huh?! You can't go against God and His plan. Who Jah blesses, no man can curse. My faith and my energy is stronger than any hate that can come my way. I want to sincerely thank you for being a no aim having cock sucker. God willing, I'll find out who you are, and God will deal with you accordingly. I'm out here changing lives, and you out here trying to take lives and failing at it, BITCH!"

"YOU CAN'T GO AGAINST GOD AND HIS PLAN"

"There is nothing noble in being superior to your fellow man; true nobility is being superior to your former self."
– Ernest Hemingway

Introduction

Between these pages are tools, and with these tools you will build a mirror. The mirror you build will reflect your favorite version of you. Mentally, you will take this mirror mindset with you everywhere: to work, job interviews, college, competitions, dates—basically into your everyday life. Your reflection will be a mixture of components that equate to your most confident self. You can mix how you feel with your best outfit on, with your most carefree state of mind, with your favorite selfie, with your most determined attitude, and/or with the feeling of your best accomplishment. My hope is that, with this reflection being with you at all times, you'll be able to ignore and eliminate insecurities, self-doubt, and self-hate. Also, over-stand that your reflection is only for you, and the more you believe what you see, the better you will feel and treat yourself, which is the reason why people will treat you better. You have to be mindful that people will treat you how you treat yourself. You'll still be you, just a more superior you, through 5 components I feel cover every aspect of life: SPIRITUAL LIFE, MENTAL LIFE, PERSONAL LIFE, HEALTHY LIFE, AND FINANCIAL LIFE.

"I was married to a state of mind, and I divorced it."
— Tariq Trotter

You In Ya Bag?

You in ya' bag? How? You haven't even captured the bag yet! I am a firm believer that whatever transpires in life is meant to be. In other words, when it comes to life, I fuck with energy. I believe whatever you speak can come into existence. It's The Law of Vibration. While working on myself, I realized speaking things into existence isn't enough. Your actions have to match what you want to see happen in your life. You know the saying, "Don't talk about it, be about it." Or, something my childhood coach would always say to me, "You gotta prove to me that you really 'bout that shit you be talking." You can't say you want to lose weight; that doesn't mean shit when you eat a bunch of Little Debbie snacks at 10 o'clock at night, laying on your back watching TV. Or that you're saving for a car but you buy designer this, designer that. Everyone has ideologies that help them balance their lives. If your actions contradict your goals then you're playing yourself, and that won't help you build the mirror.

I firmly stand on the 5 Bags of Life principle: **Spiritual**, **Mental**, **Personal**, **Health**, and **Financial**. Speaking to people has never been my thing, although I knew I was good at it. Having the ability was one thing, but I was afraid. Being the center of attention was never a goal for me. These are principles put in place by my support group (family, friends, OGs, and influencers) but not only by them. It's fair to say a lot of the principles I learned in life came from people and shit I chose not to fuck with. There's a lot of people I gladly distanced myself from because they were just not for me. I either outgrew them, or what they were into was just not my thing. That helped me build principles, which shifted the way I maneuvered. Expressed in the most confident yet humble way possible, the 5 Bags will be conducive to the evolution of a more superior you and will make you feel as ecstatic about yourself as women do when they use their favorite filters or how guys feel when they put wood Cartier glasses on. It's still you—it's just your favorite version of you.

I'm fortunate that I can share this with the masses and everyone who reads this and passes it on to a friend or associate.

This book contains gems, free game, or what me and the homies call Ragu. Although, every gem may not be for you! Everything in this book is either what helped me or those close to me make the transition to a higher level of him or herself; it also has real life analogies that helped me shift my perspective on life and myself. By putting myself in the shoes of others and determining how I would react to certain things and analyzing the possible outcomes, I was able to learn not only from my mistakes but also the mistakes of others. In other words, the **5 Bags** covers every aspect of life, and it will be the muscle behind the superior you!

As you read through this book, I hope the tools you find help you build encouragement, inspiration, guidance, and the urgency you need to make whatever aspirations you have become a reality. As the courier, my aspiration is to motivate you to "overstand." I won't use the word understand because I don't stand under anyone. The only person preventing you from becoming a better you is you! Don't be your own kryptonite.

"I'm shocked too, I'm supposed to be locked up too. You escaped what I've escaped, you'd be in Paris getting fucked up too." – Sean Carter

<u>Why 5 Bags?</u>

For my 25th birthday, I took a trip to Europe. It was one of the most surreal feelings ever. When I landed in Paris I thought to myself, "Damn! This is what Jay-Z was talking about when he said Niggas in Paris." I could finally relate to Uncle Jay in a non-struggle way. Like damn, *I'm coming from the bottom, got friends and family members that have never left the state, let alone the country. I'm in muthafuckin' Europe.* After a few days in Paris, I went to Italy. I met up with a friend from back home. He lived in a skyscraper building. I stood on the rooftop of his apartment building—yeah, his apartment was on the top of the building. Shit was dope! I remember saying to him, in probably the most vulnerable state I'd ever been in, "How can I feel this happy all the time? This is what life is supposed to feel like. I mean, I know I have to deal with reality, like death, arguments, adulthood, and whatever, but I want to feel this good all the time. Not the feeling money gives you of being "good" but the feeling of being genuinely happy. Genuine happiness should be a must in life."

We sat on the couch, watched YouTube videos, and went back and forth trying to name things that would have to align for life to be great and for us to feel great. After about five minutes of listening to my friends name things and items they'd want to possess, which were all material things, I said, "Nah man, not like that; I'm not talking about material shit, like more in refer-ence to life! There's five things. Five of em', and your bags have to be right." My boy said, "Yeah man, I need all the money!" I looked and said, "See, that's not what it's about. I can't have myself out here doing shit for money because, at some point, you gone get compromised. Money gone have you out here making a fool of yourself." There's nothing wrong with wanting the money, but you aren't going to crack the safe if you don't really enjoy what you're doing. There are five things, and they all have to align: spirituality, mentality, personal choice, and health—and they'll all help you on your financial quest.

While you consume this text, overstand it's never too late to start your journey of capturing, securing, and getting in your bags. Nor is it ever too late to get yourself on a better path. You must tell yourself that your year starts the day you begin to capture your bag. There are <u>three steps</u> to the bag culture:

**Capturing the Bag, Securing the Bag,
and Getting in the Bag.**

"Just try new things. Don't be afraid. Step out of your comfort zones and soar, alright?"
– Michelle Obama

The Phases

Step 1: Capture the Bag

To **_capture_** is to take into one's **possession** or control by **force**. *Capturing* the bag is all about the thought. It's about being able to **conceptualize** the whole scheme of things. This is when you say to yourself, there is something I want or need to do, and you plot how you will do it. It's no time to be nice. Can't be humble to an animal, and this world is the animal, the beast.

Step 2: Secure the Bag

To **_secure_** is to fix or attach something firmly so it cannot be moved or lost. *Securing* the bag is when you start to take action. This is when you now put into motion the plans you have made to change your life. This is the groundwork, the street team efforts, the extended hours in the gym, the tattooing of your blueprint into your everyday life.

Step 3: Get in the Bag

Getting in the bag is when you see satisfying rewards or changes based on the actions you have made. Getting in your bag is about staying on the correct path and remaining consistent, constantly aligning yourself with your goals. Even though this is the final step, there is no end because this is an ongoing phase of your life.

"It is better to win the peace and to lose the war."
– Robert Marley

Ready, Set...Capture!

Capturing the bag is the most salient part of the process, due to the fact that it's the beginning step. Before getting in your bag, you have to have a bag to get into. You also have to remove anything that's already in the bag to make sure you can fit as much as possible inside your bag. But what you'll be fitting into your bag is substance, not baggage, not a bunch of space fillers. With anything in life, you have to know what you want to do and how you want to do it. You must establish your plan before you set it in motion.

Let's use the game 'Capture the Flag' as an example. The objective of the game is to keep the flag as long as you can. Unfortunately, the flag is always up for grabs during the game. There's no safe area or base. No resting while you have the flag; you'll forever be the hunted. That's why it's not called 'Secure the Flag' because you'll never be able to secure it. Somebody is on your ass for it at all times. People are constantly going after the one thing you have to protect while playing the game. In the game of life, it isn't a flag you have to protect, unless you worship a flag; I'm not here to judge you if you do. You have to protect yourself and guarantee yourself growth. The bags are safe, as long as you follow your plan. No one can take away any of your bags from you. You can capture, secure, and get in all five of the bags. The only person who can take your bag from you is you. You can lose possession of the bag, if you go against the plan you have set. There are bags for everyone, so someone else capturing their bag doesn't take away the opportunity for you to capture a bag yourself.

I'm sure you're probably asking why would I take from myself? It's not as *simple* as it may seem. When you build your plan, make honesty, loyalty, trust, preparation, and readiness a part of your change. If you do something that goes against those qualities for whatever reason, that's how you metaphorically take your own bag away. It's like impeaching yourself. Anything "unbaglike" calls for a restart. Restarting doesn't mean you failed; it simply means you weren't ready to make that leap upward or had minor complications using the tools. There's no shame in that at all; keep fighting your way through, and find different ways to use your tools. Failing at something is a part of progress; it'll make you appreciate the accomplishments that much more.

Keep in mind that capturing the bag is the mental phase, the conceptualizing. Whatever thoughts or internal shifts you made to assist your change, you need to keep that thought process as long as it is working. Even when you feel like it's not, stick it through. Don't give up right away. Allowing negative thoughts to control your actions is an unbagly action. Don't be controlled by negativity. It's easier said than done, but a trick for me is always remembering that the vibrations I bring into my space can possibly, and most likely will, shift my personal space.

It's about capturing bags, not baggage. So, if there's something [some things] doesn't help you grow but you still entertain it, fuck it! Similar to how you need keys to unlock the door before entering, there are steps you need to take before getting in your bags, such as capturing and securing your bags. Baggage is dead weight. Baggage is like 'fat' on raw meat. When you're going through the heated/difficult stages of transitioning, it's like putting meat on the grill. The fat gets burned right off. That fat is your negative energy, your dead weight, your problems, your friends, and etc.

Think of the new space you would like to be in mentally, spiritually, personally, health wise, and financially as the place where unnecessary baggage is not allowed. Everyone wants to be *in* their bag, yet not everyone takes the time to remove the baggage, so they can get into their bag. You ever see women with the biggest bag, whether it's Walmart or Louis Vuitton, with threads thinning from the bag and wear and tear eating away at the material of the bag. That's the baggage you don't want in your life. Think of the snack crumbs at the bottom of the bag as bullshit, trash friendships, and situations you don't need. In every way, shape, and form baggage is a setback that blocks the outcome of your grind. If you entertain it, it'll block all your blessings. No matter what luck you believe in or what God you serve, I'll tell you this: you don't work, you don't eat. You have to put in the work. Seems like common sense, right? Well, common sense ain't so common.

Baggage should be viewed as your enemy. Remember, the only thing that can stop you is you! Baggage is like a cancer. You can live with it, but eventually it'll become harder and harder to deal with on a daily basis. Removing the cancer is extremely painful. Cancer breaks your whole body down: you lose weight, lose your hair, lose your strength, and people also lose their confidence and faith. The amazing thing is that when you beat cancer, your hair grows back, your strength comes back, and so does your weight and your confidence. Removing baggage is similar, but when the baggage is gone, you'll be so confident in yourself that you'll be able to do things you never thought were possible. However, just because the cancer was conquered, doesn't mean it can't return. If it does return, it'll be stronger than before. Baggage is the same, and you'll have to spend more effort removing it the second time.

The securing phase is similar to a revolving door: there is no ending. Securing is when you put your thoughts into actions. When conceptualizing or manifesting the plan, you may have to go back to the drawing board—remember the sacrifices you made and reevaluate your steps. For example, as part of securing my financial bag, I knew I was supposed to be saving. I went to the casino, and of course, I lost it all. I mean, who really wins at the casino. But I couldn't even be mad. I just had to say to myself, "You knew better." I was going against the plan and the pledge I made to myself. In retrospect, I deserved to lose it all. I'm not sure what I was thinking. How could I be gambling money, knowing I was supposed to be saving money? Meanwhile, I was telling people to save money and speaking on the importance of saving, false prophesying and shit. It's the Law of Vibration that I believe controls the outcome of your baglike and unbaglike decisions. This is a similar concept to "practice what you preach," which is what I explained to you earlier about your actions having to match what you want to see happen in your life. You can see what you want by speaking it into the universe and pushing your energy in that direction and maximizing your efforts!

Getting in the bag is the philanthropic, influential, or inspirational phase. It's the step that affects your universe. It's when the people who are/were around you follow your lead. I say 'were around you because of what usually happens when you begin to change your life. Motherfuckers always take offense and distance themselves, as if you're against them. However, the "getting in the bag" phase is when those people and the people in your direct circle see your actions and begin to follow your lead. That's right; you're the leader of this journey. If you haven't been a leader before, here's your opportunity. When you're in your bag, you lead by actions not words. You don't have to say anything; your actions will speak volumes.

"We can't plan life. All we can do is be available for it."
– Lauryn Hill

The Resolution to Each Bag

- **You must decide what the bag means and what personal impact it has on you.**
  For example, with the Spiritual Bag, spirituality is something outside of you physically. It is respect and reverence for yourself and your goals. It is also supplication, a humble prayer or request. But what impact does spirituality have on you as a person? First thing you have to do when using the given tools is overstand what something means to you. If it has any direct impact on you, then decide if and how you can apply it in your everyday life.

- **Understanding that each bag, at some point, requires initial isolation.**
  How much distance can you create between yourself and your distractions? Distractions can be negativity, procrastination, doubt, envy, people, etc. However, before you separate yourself physically, you must separate yourself mentally. Before you can separate yourself mentally, you have to separate yourself emotionally. You have to tap into your energy. Everything you want to shift in your life mandates that you isolate yourself from anything or anyone hindering you from doing so.

- **You have to create a framework of obedience, and put it to the test.**
  A framework is a basic structure underlying a system (whatever bag system you set up for yourself) or concept. Obedience is compliance with an order, request, law or submission to another's authority. Do so by finding a system in which you can flourish. Put yourself on a day-to-day regimen that is realistically reachable. Within your long-term goals, set short-term goals to help keep yourself on track. This will help

prevent getting lost and not realizing what and where you went wrong. The easy way out is telling yourself that something being wrong is an excuse to not reach your goal. For example, when I'm trying to get rid of a certain habit, I work on whatever it is that triggers that habit before I attempt to just break it. You have to break down everything to its smallest denominator because doing so makes it easier to overcome. I was trying to lose weight, and it was extremely difficult because I was eating late at night. I was only eating late because I was getting in the house late, and I couldn't afford to buy food every day. So, I started going to sleep earlier, so I could wake up earlier which gave me the capability to tackle my errands earlier. Then I was able to find time to work out. Between working out and being so busy all day, sleep came easier, and I wasn't up late eating a bunch of bullshit.

- **You must institute a routine after creating that framework of obedience.**
  Remember I said short-term goals? Well, a routine is a tracker for your framework of obedience—whether it be daily reminders via text, alerts to your phone or tablet device, writing on your fridge, keeping post-it notes on your desk at work, or downloading an app—the routine keeps you on point. If you're building your credit or watching your spending habits, I recommend apps like Credit Karma and Quickbooks. If you're into crypto or stocks, you have things like Coinbase, etc. There are apps for everything: building confidence, building faith—shit, there are apps for building apps. Even for setting a reminder to set your daily alarms. Do whatever will help you work on your goals.

"Tomorrow is always another day to make things right."
– Lauryn Hill

Before we begin to use these tools, I challenge you for 30 days.

- Unfollow or remove a social media friend you don't learn or gain anything from.
- Delete or block a friend who only calls you to gossip.
- Give up an addiction and bad habit.
- Compliment/Hug/Greet at least one stranger a day.
- Look in the mirror and compliment yourself every day

"Spread love and continue life. Keep creating life, that's my message." – Miguel Orlando Collins

Spiritual Bag

Inside this bag, behold the tools that will unlock your spiritual greatness, which will consequently help you to see that the universe is strong, but your willpower is stronger. Willpower is energy plus effort. Becoming one with yourself and removing traditional and methodical ways of thinking will be beneficial to accessing the advantages of spirituality.

Spiritual Bag Tips

1. Free yourself from yourself.
2. Never be a vanity slave; always know that there is no material item that can make you whole.
3. When you catch yourself judging or hating someone, ask yourself why. Overstand different cultures. They can often teach you a lot about yourself.
4. Accept your flaws, but don't embrace them.
5. Spread love; it will make you happier. Don't be the person who's too tough to laugh or too miserable to show appreciation.

In order to unlock your Spiritual Bag, you have to overstand that, by design, humans are judgmental. We're taught certain things are important, which really aren't. On the daily, remind yourself not to be green-eyed; you should not spend your days envying peoples' lifestyles, relationships, or possessions because this is not instrumental to removing the negative light from your bag. Utilizing these tools will make you more equipped to be spiritually superior to all things that go against your morals, values, and/or principles.

The Spiritual Bag should be the first bag you aspire to capture, secure, and get in. If your spirit isn't right, then you will be easily accessible to the naysayers and "well-wishing, friendly-acting, envy-hiding snakes," as Nas says.

22

The first things that come to mind for most people when they hear the word, "spiritual" are religion and God. Spirituality has nothing to do with God or religion. I made a vow to myself not to touch on religion in this book. Religion is often a roadblock to overstanding people and learning different cultures, which will hinder your ability to leverage separate realities. It can be a form of division, as far as people and unity are concerned. Regardless of your religion or belief system, as long as you feel it's making you a better person, more power to you. This Spiritual Bag is to help you disconnect from material things and connect with yourself and others through their vibrations.

"RELIGION IS OFTEN A ROADBLOCK TO OVER- STANDING PEOPLE AND LEARNING DIFFERENT CULTURES."

"Everything you imagine is real." – Pablo Picasso

The Law

Life is going to happen, and the universe will rotate regardless. It will rotate in your favor, if you're in a favorable space. Your vibrations will control your actions, which will somewhat dictate your future. It's similar to the saying, "People fear what they don't know!" Have you ever noticed when people are ignorant to something or you call them out on their ignorance, they react aggressively with harsh words, etc. It's the fear of being exposed for not being mentally equivalent to one's peers. "Everything you want will come to you when you get in harmony with it." What exactly does this mean? It means that before you get to a place you really have been looking forward to going and you actually get out the car or when you finally enter, you randomly have this feeling of uneasiness—that's the vibration of energy. Trust your energy. That shit is what connects you to everything intangible. This helps you connect to the universe. Vibrations are what make the world with so many people in it feel like such a small place because your energies connect and gravitate you to similar interests. When you speak and believe things, they'll happen. All those words with negative connotations need to be removed from your vocabulary and mental because they're more than words—they're energy. Energy is magnetic. You attract what you put into the universe.

"I'm here, and I'm confident. You'll either see me, hear me, or feel me. But you'll know I'm here." – Maurice Eastwood

Ice Breaker

Splashism: When trying to eliminate judgement, find some sort of commonality between you and the other person, preferably commonalities that don't involve material things. You would be surprised how alike you and that person are. Finding common-alities is the easiest way to eliminate judgment. You can't find commonalities unless you converse with the person. You can't approach a person thinking because you guys have the same color shirt on that you'll be best friends, but something a lot less general like a baseball cap with the same team on it can be the entrance to the commonality that will connect you to that person. There are people in the same gangs who only have one commonality, which is sharing the same set. Depending on the situation, sometimes, that's enough.

Finding similarities isn't the easiest thing to do, but ice breakers help. Life is easier with ice breakers. I learned how to be more social as I got older by mentally creating my own ice breakers. This strategy helps me to speak in front of large groups or to speak to a person first. Why do you think, in your earlier years of school or in group interviews, they have you do ice breakers where you introduce yourself and what you like to do, play two truths and one lie, or share where you're from? The purpose is to learn who everyone is in the room. It's because icebreakers help you see there's someone in the room similar to you. So, before you do something that goes against the spiritual bag and treat someone based off what you think of them without knowing anything about them, which only adds baggage to your bag, ask yourself: "Why is it that you don't want to learn anything about this person? Why is it that I dislike this person I barely know?" Is it that they remind you of something you dislike about yourself? Is there a possibility you could have things in common? This will assist in keeping an open mind and remaining curious rather than judgmental.

In the adult world, you have about 5-8 seconds for an ice breaker. After that, any type of eye contact is just weird shit. Looking at a person for 5 seconds without saying something is creepy. Commenting on shoes, a sport cap, the weather, a reason for being in the same location, or asking a nationality question are good ice breakers. I suggest staying away from news and political topics. Again, the purpose of ice breakers is to eliminate judging each other, especially when we don't even know each other.

I strongly believe humans spend so much time judging people that we forget we've got shit we need to work on ourselves. As soon as someone makes a mistake, we judge them and say, "That could never be me." We call them stupid, until we're the 'stupid' one. A lot of people suffer from believing what they were taught, and that doesn't make them weird or wrong. They know nothing else. They believe what they were taught is the only way things should go. Even if they were to learn another way, actually acting on it is difficult at first because it isn't the norm for them. Different cultures and religions deal with things differently. They even view things one culture views as evil or wrong as the norm in their religion/culture. The best yet most extreme example I can think of is terrorists who believe that if they commit certain acts of terrorism they will die and go to heaven and receive several wives. If you don't overstand their religion, how can you tell them they are wrong?

Splashism: Are you happy with who you are? Can you look in the mirror and say, "I'm me" with confidence? Do you do everything you do with love? What's your reason for doing what you do? Is it praise? These are all spiritual bag questions. The money is going to come; don't pree that. People will speak highly of you, as long as you do what you do and do it well. Doing so will open doors for opportunities. What is your why? What motivates you on the daily? Write down your answers and analyze if your motivation comes from places you're happy with, and whether it produces the results you wish to see—if not, what changes do you think you can make, to see optimal results?

_____

_____

_____

_____

_____

_____

_____

_____

_____

_____

_____

_____

_____

_____

_____

_____

_____

_____

_____

_____

_____

_____

_____

_____

"I'm building a dream with elevators in it."
– William Leonard Roberts II

Shake Some Shit Up

When the components that make up your spiritual bag are in place, the negativity will eliminate itself from your life. I mentioned earlier about the fat burning off the meat when you put it on the grill. Yes, there will be trying times, but tough times build good character. When everything is stacked against you, the tools you possess will give you the strength to overcome it, just like you've done with every other dilemma you've had up to this point. Big steps, loud steps, and meaningful steps—Allen Iverson over Tyron Lue steps.

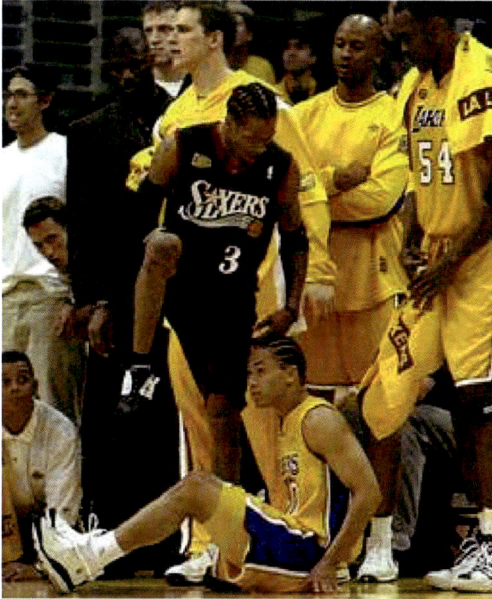

Figure 1 Allen Iverson Stepping Over Tyron Lue in NBA finals

Allen Iverson carried his team for the whole year, all the way to the NBA finals. It was modern day David vs. Goliath. The 76ers won only one game, but this picture is the most memorable part of the whole series. Allen Iverson crossed over Tyron Lue, hit the jump shot, and then took an exaggerated step over him while he was on the floor. If you're not an athlete, that's as disrespectful as someone slapping you in the face and you not being able to do anything about it. Your steps have to have substance, stomp, make some noise, shake some shit up, and cause you to exit your comfort zone. Know your worth, and know the significance and the value of the work you put in to make yourself better and to build the superior version of you.

"YES, THERE WILL BE TRYING TIMES, BUT TOUGH TIMES BUILD GOOD CHARACTER."

"Follow your inner moonlight; don't hide the madness."
— Allen Ginsberg

What They Eat Don't Make You Sh*t

Sometimes we cling to a person while on a journey because we think they are the best role model for the transition. It's admiration of the person. However, there may come a time when that person may do or say something that goes against what you once admired about them. The fact that following their steps helped you become a better version of you might make you question yourself and whether or not you've really changed. Don't question your growth! You did that. You made those changes. You fought those urges. You swallowed your pride. You found yourself. Yes, you did it—maybe with their blueprint, but it took your willpower and effort. Never give so much credit to someone else that you forget to pat yourself on the back. We're not doing easy work over here; we're trying to find the you that you aspire to be but keep getting derailed from becoming. At some point, your role model will make decisions that are not ideal for where you see yourself going. You might despise something they do, but that thing might have been what's best for them and the only way for them to walk in their truth. You can't fight their fight, and they can't fight yours. It's like hating your parents because they divorced each other, but in the marriage, they felt like prisoners. You should not hate them for making a decision for their personal happiness. You shouldn't turn your back, judge, or ridicule someone for being who they want to be.

Shared Experience: I remember talking to a friend whose mentor was cheating on his wife. His mentor helped him when he was struggling with infidelity within his marriage. When I spoke to my friend, he asked what does that mean for his relationship with his wife. First thing I told him was, "Don't let that deter you in your situation or discourage you into believing you can't be faithful. The spiritual connection you have shouldn't be with the mentor but with the mission you are on; he's just the middleman. You're your own man."

31

*"No religion, I'm just so explicit, I coexist in places
you would never know existed."
– Herbert Anthony Stevens*

<u>Divine Connection</u>

A divine connection is having a bond to something that is not materialistic. Overstand that I'm not only referring to God or a higher power. A divine connection can be a bond to anything that is sacred to you and inspires you to be a better person. There is a false belief in today's society, especially in the inner city, that being a good person is embarrassing or corny. However, let's look at this from an alternative perspective. How rewarding does it feel to pay your mother's bill for the first time? How good does it feel to make someone else you love feel good? Whether it be from buying a gift, saying something nice, or a kind gesture. How good does it feel to help a stranger who really needs it? That feeling, which correlates with materialistic good feelings, is the foundation of the spiritual bag. Just because money is not spent does not mean it isn't love. Monetary gestures should never measure the amount of love you have for something or someone.

Accept your spiritual flaws because your flaws make up who you are. You can change by working on them daily and keeping your spiritual focus. Trust the process of finding yourself during the journey. Helping people is a vital part of the Spiritual bag. Imagine if the person who was or still is the biggest influence in your life never inspired you to unlock your Spiritual bag. Imagine if you were never given a helping hand or a shoulder to lean on. Where would you be right now? Can you imagine where you'd be if that person never made you feel like achieving your dreams was possible? Especially after you've already given up on yourself. It's easy to mentally put yourself in the position of someone doing better than you, but put yourself in the position of someone doing worse than you. I guarantee you, it will change your perspective on your current situation and the way you treat people. I see it all the time when my friends come back from vacationing in developing countries or volunteering in poverty-stricken communities. They are humbled after experiencing the daily struggles of others and remember how precious their life is and how fortunate they truly are. However, once they settle back into their everyday life, it isn't the same energy. This is not a knock to them, it's just a reminder that all you have can be gone in a day. Also, some people were just born into fucked up situations. Always remember that people are important; you have to love people more than you love money— never forget that.

"A DIVINE CONNECTION CAN BE A BOND TO ANYTHING THAT IS SACRED TO YOU AND INSPIRES YOU TO BE A BETTER PERSON."

"Don't gain the world and lose your soul.
Wisdom is better than silver and gold." – Robert Marley

Revolving Door

Shared Experience: There's a lady named Mrs. Curry. Her son was my teammate in high school. I met her when I was 18-years-old, during my fifth year of high school. Yes, I did five years of high school, and no, not for sports. I was lost and doing a bunch of dumb shit, which caused some bouncing around and my family's concern for me ending up in prison or dead. Anyway, after knowing me for only one month, she took on a responsibility most wouldn't want. She opened the doors of her home to an 18-year-old nigga from the hood. That's how I would describe myself back then. I didn't know who I was, nor did I have any real idea of self. I believe I wasn't even trying to find myself because my environment confirmed I had already "made it." I made it past 16 and lived long enough to experience being 18. Life didn't have much to offer, honestly. I was in trouble at school two to three times a week for the past four years of high school. Once my environment changed by moving in with the Curry family, my actions followed suit. But back to the lady; she wanted to see me do better, off the strength of me being her son's friend. I was so lost and selfish that I felt as if she took me in to keep her son closer to her. I assumed she thought if the people in her son's life are around her, then her son would be too. In other words, *if his friends aren't out doing anything wild then he won't be either.* I often refer to Mrs. Curry as my angel on earth, if you believe in that type of thing. I would often wonder, "Why me? What's in it for her?" If I ever got in trouble at school, she had no problem hitting me with, "C'mon, you can't do that." If I had a bad game, she'd tell me I played like crap. If the referees were on the bullshit at one of my games, she'd tell them. She always celebrated my accomplishments as if they were her own, and when I was in a jam, there she was once again.

When people don't give a fuck about you, they don't care to right your wrongs; you'll know they don't care at all when they let you carry on with your foolishness. As my coach would always say, "As long as I'm saying something that means I care. When I stop

"A single word can change our reality. And that word is Yes."
– Kwame Alexander

Things to be Mindful of when Capturing the Spiritual Bag

1. Add prayers or meditation to your weekly/daily routine. It doesn't have to be on a knee or in a church, but speak positivity outward and wish blessings for those around you.
2. You'll never be able to unconditionally love anyone until you love yourself.
3. Embrace others; hug people!
4. Whatever higher power you believe in, always remember they love you more than you love yourself.
5. No item should ever mean more to you than a person. Don't be a vanity slave. As Robert Marley once said, "The greatness of a man is not in how much wealth he acquires, but in his integrity and his ability to affect those around him positively."[2]

---

2   (Account 2012)

correcting you, that's when you know I'm done with you." I know you're probably wondering how this relates to the Spiritual Bag, but simmer down. Let me connect the dots.

The older I got, the more I became knowledgeable enough to overstand that Mrs. Curry had already captured and secured her Spiritual bag. She secured her Spiritual bag when she cared for my success and well-being more than I cared for my own. In the simplest terms, she saved my life. The impact she has had in my life is a feeling I now aspire to give someone else. This is what I mean by "getting in the bag" spiritually. When someone is in their bag, their aura is powerful enough to pull you into their world or mindset. When you're in your bag, you will then be able to affect many people by affecting one person. This is what Mrs. Curry did for me. One of the reasons why it's so easy for me to help people is because she has helped me, and I hope the people I help do the same for someone else. I look at helping people as a small family tree with many branches. The people I help she'll never know about it, but she's one of the roots of that tree in my life, and there's a root to her tree I don't know about. That's what keeps the world growing, yet keeps it so small and always revolving.

"WHEN PEOPLE DON'T GIVE A FUCK ABOUT YOU, THEY DON'T CARE TO RIGHT YOUR WRONGS."

*"No one knows my struggle, they only see the trouble.
Not knowin' it's hard to carry on when no one loves you."*
– Tupac Shakur

The Streets Don't Love You

For my readers who are in the streets, never believe your prayers aren't working. Certain things may have occurred causing you to find yourself caught up in the streets, selling drugs, using drugs, robbing, stealing, and putting in work—sometimes, it's just the way the cards are dealt. I'm sure you want to do better but don't know how, or you're so deep in that you feel stuck. Keep your faith! Don't make excuses, make changes.

Never allow anyone to tell you your prayers don't work. That's bullshit. Speak it into the universe, follow it up with effort and energy. Think about it: you're in the streets every day, how is it possible that you dodged those cops, those bullets, the enemies, or made it out of that tight situation when you thought it was over for you? Sounds like a power working for you not against you; it sounds like good energy. That power is your spirit, the energy of prayer. We all pray whether it's with eyes open or closed, on two knees with hands raised, or after doing 80 in a 65 zone and seeing a cop.

Splashism: The reality is, every time we step outside of our home it could be our last time seeing our family, regardless of what we do for a living. It's true that within certain lifestyles the risk of not seeing tomorrow is amplified. When you're fucking with the streets more times than none, the end result will be prison or death. Smoking and/or selling drugs can't stop the Spiritual bag or its blessings. The prayers or the spiritual presence from your loved ones is what's getting you out of those jams. Don't let anyone tell you that you don't have a chance because you're in a gang, caught a case, did some dirt, been to jail, or sell drugs. For some people, a gang affiliation saved their lives, sheltered them when no one else would, and fed them when no when else could. I say all this to say regardless of your situation, you are never too far from securing the Spiritual bag. Spirituality doesn't mean religion, but I do believe it involves believing in a higher power outside of yourself.

It's people like you, who turned their lives around and have the biggest impact on people without spending a dime. However, don't allow doubt to be your excuse. Let it be your motivation. At the end of your journey, you won't be who you are now; you'll be who you are currently aspiring to be. No drug dealer wants to sell drugs forever. No killer wants his kids growing up busting guns like him. That ain't gangsta!

"KEEP YOUR FAITH! DON'T MAKE EXCUSES, MAKE CHANGES."

*"As gang members, as young dudes in the streets...
we're the efect of a situation. We didn't wake up
and create our own mind-state and our environment.
We adapted our survival instincts." -Ermias Asghedom*

When you get in the bag, overstand you're now the leader of a lifestyle for your followers, friends, family, and most important-ly yourself. Figure out what will motivate you to continue your quest to greatness.

What you consume consciously or subconsciously on a daily basis, shouldn't make you question yourself; if it does, your spirit is vulnerable to everything. You should protect your spirit and energy the same way you'd protect your most prized posses-sion. The goals you've set for yourself are easy to lose track of if your spirit is accessible, leaving room for jealousy to control your thought process and for envy to control your heart. Being knowl-edgeable of that fact will put you in position to clearly recognize your own irrational unbaglike behaviors.

Being spiritually intact is also not allowing material items to overcome your soul. If you're an adult and want to fight because you got your shoes stepped on, someone in the house drank the last of your damn apple juice, or you're spending your last on designer to be socially accepted, then you're lost, and I'd advise you to find yourself quickly. Don't worship that shit. In reality, shit loses value once you purchase it. Instead of being a vanity slave, focus on things that cleanse your heart and help you see things as half full as opposed to half empty. This keeps you completely optimistic. Pursue things that will affect the world when you're no longer here in the physical form. That's why living knowing that you're laying a blueprint is more important than any amount of likes on social media or any amount of cars and jewelry.

Another tool to securing your Spiritual bag is finding out what makes you a better person. Capturing the spiritual bag is simply being mindful enough to realize that you previously put your faith, hope, love, or motivation in the wrong place.

Tell yourself it's time to make a change. Remember the capturing phase is just conceptualizing. Once you realize your first objective from that point should be to focus on making less unbaglike decisions.

"BEING SPIRITUALLY INTACT IS ALSO NOT ALLOWING MATERIAL ITEMS TO OVERCOME YOUR SOUL."

"Vacation to Haiti, it nearly broke my heart. Seeing kids starve,
I thought about my Audemar."
– William Leonard Roberts II

Spiritual Bag Questions

1. Are you materialistic?
2. Do you love yourself?
3. Do you believe in a higher power?
4. How easily controlled is your energy?
5. Who is the root and branches of your tree?

"What you gonna do? Lift up your head and keep moving, or let the paranoia haunt you?" – Kendrick Duckworth

Mental Bag

The tools inside the Mental bag will assist you with clarity, peace of mind, transparency, and unveiling a more confident you. Conceptualizing your weaknesses and accepting that every day is an opportunity for growth will guide you to a mental space of what I refer to as 'unfuckwithableness," which is knowing what you want and having the confidence and demeanor of a person who is untouchable and overstanding that the mental is critically essential. So we thinketh, so it can be.

Mental Bag Tips:

1. Never let someone's opinion dictate your day, especially if they're not paying you.
2. Take care of your mental.
3. Open a book, and challenge yourself.
4. Overstand that nothing lasts forever, so learn what you can from who/what you can.
5. Only you can be you.

"They say money rules the world, you can't pay God with it." – Robert Williams

Placebo Effect

I'm sure you've been called many different things by people close to you and people who don't know shit about you. But, who the fuck cares? I've been told I was a thug, a thief, a killer, a bum, a bitch ass nigga, a bully, inadequate—basically, everything you can think of. But I didn't let the titles they assigned to me control the perception I had of myself. You have to equip yourself with the mental tools to avoid being manipulated into being a victim of what I call the Placebo Effect. A placebo is prescribed for the psychological benefit to the participant, rather than the physiological effect. A placebo is basically a mental "cure." The cure does not put anything in your body that is not already there. What the placebo does is make you think you are aiding whatever illness or shortcoming you may have, when in reality it ain't doing shit. The cure was already within you, but the lack of confidence and awareness of self does not allow you to overstand that you already possess these mental tools. The 'Placebo Effect' is when you start to question yourself based on the label others use to refer to you. You have to know and believe you can conquer whatever is stacked in front of you. There is never a time where you should quit because you feel the odds are stacked against you. Shit, the odds of you being here in the physical form proves you are an overcomer. Out of 100 million other sperm cells, you're the only one who made it. I call this the Sperm Count Theory. You started your life as a winner. You won before you were even born. You were the winning sperm to make it to the egg and survive in the womb. You only get one life to live, make the most of every day, and make meaningful decisions. When you begin to fall victim to the Placebo Effect remember, YOU ARE THE SPERM THAT MADE IT.

No matter how successful you are, people will slander your name and pray for your downfall. Let me say this again, *no matter how successful you are people will slander your name and pray for your downfall.* Overstand that reality will strengthen you with the mental tool of blocking out baggage. Think of a person you love and respect. How many people dislike that person or have something negative to say about him or her? Even if it doesn't reflect the version of them that you know, there is no one in this world who is liked by everyone. No matter your net worth or skill set, the world will never collectively love you. It's not a realistic aspiration, to be liked by everyone. You can look at your favorite celebrity's social media page and find endless negative remarks in the comments, even if their post is positive. Let's use Floyd Mayweather for example. He has never lost a professional fight in his whole career, and people still have negative things to say about him as a boxer, not because of his boxing skills but because of his personal life and the perception they create. This goes to show, no matter what you do and how well you do it, negative remarks are bound to be made. The toxic things people say about others are simply a reflection of their bitter selves. Never let what's said about you become who you see when looking at yourself in the mirror.

Splashism: Use the Sperm Count Theory as a cheat code to become the winner in every situation that seems insurmountable. Thrive off of it. If you are wondering what there is to thrive off of, it isn't hate. Hate is mental. Everyone always says, 'Hate is my motivator.' The question I always ask myself is how do you know it's hate coming from someone and not just constructive criticism? How do you tell the difference? Is what is being said the painful truth? If so, that's not hate. Thrive off of what could be and should be to you. Instead of saying, "I'm gonna prove this person wrong, cause they're hating." Why not just prove yourself right?

Reflect and think about the words people have used to describe you. Decide whether or not they were accurate to your actions at the time. Record your thoughts.

_____

_____

_____

_____

_____

_____

_____

_____

_____

_____

_____

_____

_____

_____

_____

_____

_____

_____

_____

_____

_____

_____

_____

_____

_____

_____

_____

_____

If you could not find one thing to write proceed to "Nobody Worried 'Bout Yo Ass" and revisit this section.

"Everybody's got opinions on the way you're livin,' but see, they can't fill your shoe." – André Lauren Benjamin

Nobody Worried 'Bout Yo Ass

You will have 'haters' in every area of your life. However, it is problematic if you start believing that everyone is hating on you. Everyone is entitled to their opinion, no matter how foolish their opinion is to you. Instead of feeling bad for yourself, check yourself to see if their opinions are accurate versus delusional. If you believe everyone is always against you, what actually might be happening is reality and your insecurities sinking in that the quality of your work, product, loyalty, or skill level isn't as good as you want it to be. Do you remember when mom bought you those knock off kicks and the off-brand clothes and kids would make fun of you? You'd call them haters, but deep down, you knew your clothes were whack. You'd call them haters just to get them off your case, so you could feel better about yourself. Instead of making everyone out to be your enemy, listen to what they say. Master the art of picking sense from nonsense.

It's fair to say hate isn't the best motivator. In reality, if you're dwelling on the 'hate' more so than self-doubt, your real issue is internal, which means you need to revisit the Spiritual bag. People who throw the word 'hate' around loosely may be fighting a feeling of failure. The feeling that they aren't as qualified or equipped as the competition is beginning to sink in, and it's hard to accept. Instead of working on themselves, the first thing they do is say someone is hating on them. When an adult says they have haters, it always throws me for a loop. I feel like sometimes it's more so mental. Haters in your high school days? Yeah, maybe. I guess that makes sense. But once you're out of college and aging, no one cares about your accomplishments, clothing, car, kids, or any of that stuff—unless what they're saying about you is accurate, why let it bother you? Just know, someone is always watching you and judging what you are doing.

Lastly, you have people who will bet their last dollar that they have all these social media 'haters'—don't be this person. You have to ask yourself, "How do I know I have haters, especially if the people 'hating' are behind my back or on the other side of the social media app?" The only people close enough to knowingly be a hater are your friends or close associates, which we're going to talk about it in the Personal bag. If telling yourself you have haters works for you, then more power to you. Nonetheless, be careful so you don't put yourself on a mental 'high horse' and block the wrong person out by accusing someone with legitimate criticism of "hating." If the person matters enough or what they say matters enough, take heed to what is said, and dissect it. If a bunch of people say the same thing, there's some truth to it. Let your ambition to be great motivate you, not hate. When you reach one goal, use that accomplishment to push you to reach your next goal. That's what separates the Serena Williams, Nipsey Hussle, Marcus Garvey, and Beyonce types of the world from everyone else. What people say about you should never be the deciding factor to any of your actions or plans. For every person who thinks you're a waste of sperm, there's a person who thinks you're God's gift to the world. The people who see the glass as half empty will either think of you as a weirdo or a genius for looking at it as half full. People will forever be unsatisfied, and it is not your job to satisfy them. Removing your ego will help with deciding whether someone is hating on you or giving constructive criticism.

We are only dealing with identifying the 'haters' that are in your immediate circle because none of the other 'haters' matter. The way I differentiate criticism versus hate is by actions and words. You can identify a hater when they use words like 'lil' to acknowledge your accomplishments. For instance, I see you with your "lil Honda," with your "lil chain," etc. Secondly, if they use "**you**, I, and **me**" more than they use "**us** and **we**." The use of "we" and "us" show they are in your corner and want to see you win. Anyone I consider a friend has shown happiness to a level where it was clear they were happy for "us."

- Why not just block the social media friends whom you feel hate on you?
- Analyze your immediate circle, and determine if any of them are your actual haters.
- If you are honest with yourself, then nothing anyone says to you should matter.
- You're not always right.

The Mental bag is about envisioning what you wish to see come to fruition, which I referred to before as the capturing phase. Think of your Mental bag as your third eye. The third eye is known as the gateway to higher consciousness. It is located in the same spot as the pineal gland in your brain. Pineal gland is at the geometric midpoint of our brain and is intimately associated to how our body receives light. It even modulates our wake-sleep patterns. The third eye is often referred to as the "Seat of the Soul,"[3] so when I say, "see it," I mean mentally. The third eye is already there, you just have to tap into it—in other words, open your eyes. Oops! I mean mind! Adversities will stack against you, and others will expect you to break. The baggage will feel too heavy; however, no such thing is true. No baggage or intangible weight can be too heavy. It's either heavy or it isn't. There is no such thing as too cold, too hot, too weak, too small. *Too* is another word for *can't*, and the use of either signifies that you have mentally defeated yourself before attempting to defeat it. It's critical that you have a plan in place to help you reach your mental destination. Realistically, you're one of two things: built tough enough for the trials and tribulations or just not built at all. Some people have breakdowns, and some people have breakthroughs. Some people get in their bag, and some people let the baggage block them. Your biggest threat to people is your Mental bag. If you believe something intangible can hold you down, you will forever be defeated. Your thoughts, your friends, your current relationships, and your lifestyle are all examples of intangible barriers. Those aren't physical barriers, as opposed to being cuffed to a bed or stuck under a rock. The third eye is a tool only some unlock but a tool we all possess.

"THE THIRD EYE IS KNOWN AS THE GATEWAY TO HIGHER CONSCIOUSNESS."

3   (THIRD EYE PINECONES 2018)

"I never learned hate at home, or shame. I had to go to school for that." – Richard Gregory

Self-Love is Lit

Self-love is amazing. It consists of fun, well-being, physical and mental health, emotional awareness, therapy, and pampering. Self-love is all about making yourself feel appreciated, noticed, and like a King/Queen. The first step of self-love is realizing you can always love yourself more. Self-love is a process that requires patience, attention to detail, and the determination to find mental peace.

THERAPY WITH A THERAPIST IS FUCKING LIT. Seeing a therapist is often frowned upon and looked at as weakness. If seeing a therapist is weakness, then we should all be some weak ass people. Participating in some type of therapy shows your strength, your self-love, and dedication to being a more superior you. In other words, going to therapy shows that you give a fuck about yourself. For me, it brings a certain level of peace. It's a place where I can sit and talk to someone with unbiased feedback. You will know your therapist is the right one when you do not feel like you're pouring your heart out to a stranger. No matter who you are, you need to talk to someone. Therapists won't ever have all the answers, they're not psychic. You are the one with the answers; therapy just helps you answer a lot of your own questions. Having a therapist is like life being a final exam and having access to the cheat sheet. A certain amount of transparency is unlocked with therapy. Honesty and therapy go hand-in-hand; you have to be able to walk in your truth, which will make speaking about your life easier once you overstand that nothing can be undone but that everything can be fixed. Seeing small changes to your thought process and reactions to the bullshit life throws at you session-by-session is very fulfilling. I would at least suggest trying therapy before knocking it. I mean, think of all the things you have tried that are in no way beneficial to you being a more superior you.

- What's the reason you don't go to therapy?
- Do you know anyone who goes to therapy?

Write your reason below, and read it to yourself aloud.

_____

_____

_____

_____

_____

_____

_____

_____

_____

_____

_____

_____

_____

_____

_____

_____

_____

_____

_____

_____

_____

_____

_____

_____

_____

_____

After you have written you reason(s), do you still feel it's legit-imate to not attend therapy? If your answers contain, "There's nothing wrong with me," or "I already know what's wrong with me. Why do I need a therapist to tell me?" then you need ther-apy! If you don't want to go to therapy, talk to a friend. Talk to a mirror. Talk to anyone besides the voices in your head.

I need you to think of how you meditate and do exactly that. Take 5 minutes and meditate the best way you know how. Go ahead, put the book down, and meditate. Whether it's listening to a song, praying, chanting, simply gazing, put the book down and do so.

Initial isolation is like a reset button for the brain that's essential to you being on top of your shit. You have to know when your brain and body are due for a recharge. Sleeping is important, fueling your body is important, and meditation is important. If you are a person of very limited time, a simple pause to take time for deep in and out breathing is beneficial. Some days, meditation might be an hour of pure quietness. No phone, no distractions, just you and your thoughts or even a little music. The better you get at meditating, the better you'll get at escaping the negative energies, which will ultimately limit the effect that intangible things have on you.

There are many forms of meditation; it's important to find out what meditation works best for you. I advise that meditation not need any component other than self. Meaning, the component should not be smoking, drinking, or any sort of spending activity. Things like walking, taking deep and exaggerated breaths, lay-ing/sitting in quietness, or even screaming can be a therapeutic form of meditation. Music is a great component to add. Another thing that works for me is writing in my journal. Personally, I write or talk to myself to avoid reacting to certain people and certain behaviors. Afterward, I go back to read and analyze if the way I reacted was me being in control of my actions or me allowing the situation to control me. This helps me a lot with learning how to be rational and to separate myself emotionally from certain things. No, it's not about being perfect, it's about a daily progres-sion of controlling emotion and controlling what gets you riled up. Finding humor in things that aren't really funny is another way I avoid being controlled by words and actions of people who

I think should jump off a fucking cliff. Back to meditation though: there's apps that teach you to meditate, YouTube channels, books, and social media pages dedicated solely to meditating. Lastly, if none of that works, find whatever it is that makes you happy, and do it a lot.

Meditation for me is:

- Laying on the floor with the lights and music off and my phone on silent.
- Listening to albums that put me in a peaceful mood or mixing Bob Marley with Future or mixing Lauryn Hill with Sza.
- Closing my eyes and taking deep breaths, no matter where I am.
- Squeezing a stress ball.
- Doing Yoga.
- Talking to myself aloud is my favorite.

List 5 ways you will meditate:

1. _____
2. _____
3. _____
4. _____
5. _____

"He who seeks knowledge begins with humbleness."
– Mark Myrie

One Step at a Time

Instead of dwelling on what you think you can't do, figure out ways to accomplish what you want to do. Create small goals: daily, weekly, monthly, and yearly. The reason for this is that everything in life takes time. You have to have patience and let things evolve and grow. Patience is often an overlooked factor; the more patience you have, the greater the outcome. The greatness you achieve will create a hunger that can only be filled by an accomplishment of that same magnitude. If you run into a roadblock or you fail, it's okay. When you get up, you'll be sharper, better, and stronger than the last time. Nothing can hold you back from being as great as you aspire to be.

Shared Experience: My college years were the most dreadful. Not a bone in my body looked forward to class or campus. The ultimate motivation was the promise I made to my grandmother and mother who spent months begging me to go to college because they didn't want me trying to hustle and finesse my way through life. My grandmother and I are super close; disappointing her would've done something to my soul and mind that I wouldn't be able to forgive myself for. That's what motivated me—through rain, sleet, or snow—to get my ass up and go to class. When I didn't study and had to cheat, I told myself, "If you ain't cheating, you ain't trying." That was my fake "*by any means necessary*" approach. I knew I had to cheat and be as discreet as possible because getting caught would mean being kicked out of college, money down the drain, and debt up to my neck, not to mention disappointing my Grandma.

On the day of graduation, when I saw that smile and felt the energy from my whole family (mother and grandma specifically), that was the first time I felt something money can never replace. That's a feeling that has motivated me to this day. It's a feeling I've been chasing. The moral of the story isn't about cheating to get by but rather that sometimes you have to do things you don't want to do and you are going have to find a way to get done what needs to get done. Although it isn't the path you wish to travel, it'll still get you to your destination. The original plan you had might've been easier and shorter, but sometimes shortcuts aren't always the best route to take. My 8th grade Math teacher would always tell me, "The quickest way from point A to Point B is always a straight line," and now I see what he meant: stop trying to go around your problems, and go through them.

Motivation built on aspirations are often the best because it comes from an empty space in you that needs to be filled. It makes the process enjoyable, and the tough times endurable! For the next big step you take, you will want to find that feeling again—the motivation. The motivation to be Jordan spraying champagne and puffing a cigar, Usain Bolt taunting his opponents during the race, Snoop Dogg thanking himself for all his accomplishments, or Puff Daddy in the "If I Ruled the World Video."

"Death is not the greatest loss in life.
The greatest loss is what dies inside while still alive.
Never surrender."
– Tupac Shakur

The Hate U Give Little Infants Fucks Everybody

"The seeds that you plant grow and blow up in your face"[4]
- Tupac. The Mental bag is about being secure and
solidified in yourself. There are seeds planted *by* you and seeds
planted *in* you. These seeds either grow to their maximum potential or never bloom. These seeds are a part of your spiritual
and mental structure.

We all have seeds planted for us and in us by others: parents,
teachers, friends, and society. The seeds planted make you
think you are great, you are poor, you are
missing out, you will never become anything, your
existence is a mistake, you shouldn't love yourself, or you love
yourself too much. The seeds make you think you have too
many friends or that you prove your importance through material
achievements or possessions.

But those seeds grow and blossom and when they do, BOOM!
That boom can either be who they said you were or who you tell
yourself you are. That boom is the outcome. The blossoming of
those seeds doesn't have to be the measure of success.

What they blossom *into* is the byproduct.

Be sure you are able to handle the byproduct of the seed you
planted.

---

4   (Tupac explains thug life 2007)

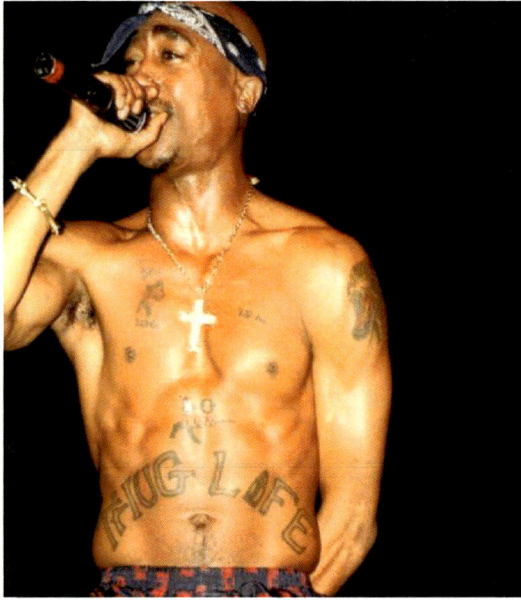

THUG LIFE stands for The Hate U Give Little Infants Fucks Everybody[5]—as infamously tattooed on Pac's stomach. Pac felt the government painted a picture of minorities in America as thugs, goons, hoodlums, scum, unruly, and the list goes on. He felt the seeds planted in minorities were to keep minorities mentally imprisoned as people who would work and continue to work. He felt that for every positive seed planted, there are thousands of negative seeds being planted. Tupac shook up the world by using all the seeds planted to hold people of color back and using every negative stereotype about Blacks as a weapon for elevation and liberation, and he reminded you of it in every song, video, or performance when you'd see him with his shirt off or open. What better way to disrupt the seed planters than having THUG LIFE tattooed right under the AK 47 with 50 niggas written to represent the 50 states. If that wasn't enough, he replaced the 'I' in LIFE with a bullet. For all the wrongdoings, injustice, and violence against Blacks, he reminds you of it every time you see and hear his voice. Without ever retaliating physically, you can still affect the seed planter mentally. This is what being in your bag is about—using the tools of opposition to elevate yourself and whomever you're fighting for.

---

5   (Tupac explains thug life 2007)

Being in your bag is about using those seeds that people planted to tell you what you are and when you can and can't blossom and becoming the seed that blossoms not only in the garden, but in the fucking concrete. It takes ambition and fight. Anything can grow through a crack in the concrete, but can you blossom? That is the question. Capture *that* bag. Secure *that* bag. Get in *that* bag. When you do blossom, use your full capabilities to change the narrative and use everything we have conversed about so far in the Mental bag to become 'unfuckwithable.'

"WITHOUT EVER RETALIATING PHYSICALLY, YOU CAN STILL AFFECT THE SEED PLANTER MENTALLY."

"It is much easier to show compassion to animals. They are never wicked." – Haile Selassie

You Hurt You

Splashism: My goal with the Mental bag is to help you to become more realistic and logical. When you view things from that standpoint, others will say, "Why you gotta be so negative?" or "Why you so hurt; who hurt you?" The answer may not be external. Is it fair to say you can hurt yourself? Can you be your own nightmare? Can you get in your own way? Yes, that is very possible.

If you expose yourself to something abnormal or rare and tell yourself that is the feeling that you want on a daily basis, you're creating a level of expectation that you won't be able to reach, which can cause unhappiness and frustration. For example, you're in a relationship, in which you're expected to be loyal, but you go out and spend time with someone else or have sex with someone else who's a little more active during intercourse. They also let you talk to them however during a regular conversation, which makes you feel in charge and feeds your ego. Fast forward to when you're with your significant other, their lack of submissiveness or their demand for respect during a conversation might rub you wrong or irritate you. Shit, if they breathe too hard, you get pissed. Is it really them irritating you? Or is it what you let yourself get accustomed to? They didn't change and neither did you, but what you did was allow someone else's energy to come in, spoil you, and disrupt your everyday space. Their energy overpowered your mind. You had no issues with their ways before letting someone change your expectations. Now your expectations are altered because one person did something for you, and now you feel the person you're in a relationship with should also. You completely disregard the leaps they've made to become who you have been asking them to become. Instead, you want what you have tasted, which has now become the new goal for you. Unfortunately, the only way to reach that goal is to get it outside of your situation. Another example of this would be, every time you go to a basketball game, you sit in the upper deck with your significant other. Another guy takes you to a game at this same arena, but the tickets are for courtside seats. Now, when you go back to the same place for another game, you don't want to be there because the seats aren't courtside. Little do you know, they won those tickets when you went courtside. The guy who takes you all the time is spending money for the tickets, but that isn't good enough anymore because you've allowed yourself to get used to an unrealistic lifestyle at this point. In other words, "Congrats, you played yourself."

This falls in your Personal bag, Spiritual bag, and Mental bag. It's Personal because you put yourself in the situation to do nothing but play yourself and fuck up your happiness. It's Spiritual because you allowed them to interrupt your mood and actions; you showed you're weak in many ways, bought dreams, and showed that you'll probably fuck up the same way the next time something that meets the eye comes around. It's Mental because you have to overstand the predicaments you're putting yourself in and what you're jeopardizing. So yes, someone can hurt you—but you can also hurt yourself by blocking your blessings. Before you eliminate something or someone out of your space, be sure of your decisions. The grass might be greener on the other side but shit, that grass might look so good because it's really turf.

How often do you allow yourself to let people/actions affect your reality? Is your reality often affected by more than one thing? Would you consider yourself gullible?

_____

_____

_____

_____

_____

_____

_____

_____

_____

_____

_____

_____

_____

_____

_____

_____

_____

_____

_____

_____

_____

_____

_____

_____

_____

"If you sharing your success and not your struggles you a fool."
– Ermias Asghedom

Splashism: Do you ever feel like you're failing or waiting for the perfect opportunity to appear, the "right time"? The reality is you'll never know when it's the right time until you make a decision and find out it was the wrong time.

You can attempt to convince yourself that a certain job is for you or that a certain person is for you, and you'll probably believe that until you're no longer working there or involved with that person. Then you're like, "That wasn't for me" or "What the fuck was I thinking?" You can sit around waiting for perfect, but perfect will not appear. We often forget to factor in growth, wisdom, and knowledge. Our own growth or wisdom may make us ask, "What was I thinking?" Growth and wisdom can't be taught, they come from experience. You ever see those Facebook flashbacks and read some of your posts or see a throwback picture and say, "What the fuck?" or "Oh my God!"—yeah, that's growth!

Growth is finding yourself after a hurtful relationship, a life-changing scenario or a tough time, helping you to build confidence moving forward. You learn how to ride your bike not only because you have fallen but because you learned that falling hurts, so you figure out how to avoid it. Nonetheless, don't be afraid to fall. Let go of fears, and let life help you find you. Every time you get up you'll bounce back tougher. Those scars you get from falling on your life journey will heal. Some scars will need band aids, some will need stitches, some falls might even need surgery because something is broken. But when it heals, it heals stronger! That is exactly how you'll heal and bounce back from trials: stronger!

Speaking of consumption more generally, one of the most obtainable things in our culture is also one of the worst things for you to consume: social media. Instagram, Facebook, and Twitter are places where you see how people want you to think they live. Social media can be very useful, but it can be a deterrent to your own internal development because you catch yourself saying, "I need to get my shit together" and do this and that because you see someone doing what you think you should be doing. If it takes up time and fills you with false assumptions, then you damn sure aren't ready to be a boss. You should back away from social media, and take time to be alone. Find yourself instead of finding out what others are doing.

"THOSE SCARS YOU GET FROM FALLING ON YOUR LIFE JOURNEY WILL HEAL."

"I think I'm the best at everything that I do. I may be biased because it's me. But if you ask me that, that's what I'm going to tell you." – Cameron Giles

Power of Both Pressures

Splashism: The pressure of proving the naysayers wrong vs. the pressure of proving your supporters right is something we all go through. Don't let what naysayers say break you. On the other hand, don't let what your supporters say about you pressure you into being something other than what you desire. Find the middle ground. You're going to be in certain places in your life where people make you feel like you just don't have that "it" factor. You'll also be in certain places in life where people are expecting more than you can offer. Don't get caught up in the pressures of either. This is why you live your life for yourself, and if you don't, you should start. Often, we get so caught up in everyone else that we forget about ourselves, allowing people to live vicariously through us while also striving to prove people wrong at the same time.

Shared Experience: I started playing basketball at the age of ten. I played with and against players I was better than, who would also tell me how "garbage" I was. People told me I would be a professional one day, whether you know it or not, a simple compliment sometimes comes with weight you think people want you to live up to. Never would they ask what I wanted to do with my life. They'd only told me what they thought would be best for me to do. On a daily basis, I was caught between trying to prove the naysayers wrong, while at the same time trying to prove my supporters right. I never actually took the time to think about what I truly wanted for me.

As a kid, I believed my success in life was limited to the realm of entertainment, such as being an athlete, rapper,

or selling whatever drug was lit at the time. I wasn't exposed to alternative paths to success, whether those paths were through art, being a doctor, an engineer, or even a teacher. I didn't know anyone who was in any of those professions, so I didn't think it was a realistic expectation for me. I'd say, "When I grow up, I will be a doctor," but that was because that's what I saw on TV. I also had to learn not to allow the peer pressure from my supporters to cause me to commit to something I was unhappy with.

The moral of the story is, know when it's time to hang up a certain dream or know when you're not into something and only doing it to please someone. Don't waste you prime chasing what you don't want. Instead, take that time and build toward what it is that your heart really desires.

"THIS IS WHY YOU LIVE YOUR LIFE FOR YOURSELF, AND IF YOU DON'T, YOU SHOULD START."

Take a second to sit back and reflect on how often you do things just to prove people wrong and/or to prove people right? What good does it do to you? How does it make you feel?

_____

_____

_____

_____

_____

_____

_____

_____

_____

_____

_____

_____

_____

_____

_____

_____

_____

_____

_____

_____

_____

_____

_____

_____

_____

_____

_____

_____

"My greatest pain in life is that I will never be able to see myself perform live." – Kanye West

Kanye

Splashism: Say what you want about Kanye West. I know a bunch of people who say Kanye is brainwashed. Some people even joke that the movie *Get Out* is about him, that he sold his soul, and that he's mentally weak. I don't think this is the case at all, but that's not for me to decide. When it comes to the bags, we deal with facts rather than opinions. The fact is, Kanye did something most guys run from: he got married to his children's mother. He married and started a family with the same woman who he has children with. Not a regular everyday woman—a mogul, slander target, a woman who has a sex tape all over the internet. A woman who gets bashed for the amount of guys she's dated. A woman who comes from a family that gets accused of only wanting to date rich, Black celebrities. She's portrayed to have been out here doing promiscuous things with multiple Black athletes and celebrities. 'Ye even talks about it in his music: "I bet me and Ray J would be friends, if we ain't love the same bitch. Yeah, he might have hit it first. Only problem is, I'm rich." A lot of my associates—both White and Black—don't even want to talk to a girl who is known by too many guys. Kanye also went on a two-year long rant about getting his YEEZY brand some respect. He believed his brand would out sell all the major brands. None of the business players in positions of power wanted to help him. He was so mentally locked in on the situation that people started to say drugs were getting to him. Maybe they were; maybe they weren't. I don't know what it feels like to have so many people bashing you for wanting to follow your dreams. However, the fact that he mentally locked in and never lost focus of the bigger picture is admirable. For someone of such celebrity status to go through that much slander and public ridicule for believing in himself and STILL find a way to come out on top shows why being in tune with yourself, believing in yourself, and unlocking the Mental bag is an asset to fully unveiling a more superior you. He never allowed the naysayers to stop him. His mental toughness and determination led to the most coveted sneaker release ever from a non-athlete. First chance 'Ye got to show his ass to his doubters he did so in his music by saying, "Hold up, I ain't trying to stunt, man. But these Yeezys jumped over the Jumpman" in reference to selling more than the Jordan brand. The moral of the story is to stick to your plan and have patience, drive, belief in self, like Kanye. Most importantly if you get told no ten times, go for the eleventh.

Confidence is a major factor. It's a thin line between confidence and cocky and when you feel like you're the only one fighting for what you believe in. You are going to have to walk that line. You have to have enough confidence in yourself to fight the fight. Stand on your dreams, build your cloak to avoid people from coming in. The risk of getting blacked-balled when you actually have shit to lose is something you have to decide if you are willing to do. You can always pretend that nothing is wrong, but insecurities stick out, people notice them. The more you try to camouflage, the more evident it becomes. It stands out, and I mean really stands out, like wearing Easter colors to a funeral where everyone is wearing all black.

"I don't stress out, nigga. Poke my chest out, nigga.
Weight on my shoulder, bring the best out, nigga."
– Ermias Asghedom

Stress

Splashism: Do not let stress kill you. STRESS IS NOT REAL. Actually, stress is as real as you make it. Inhale, exhale, and say it aloud, "I control my stress." Again, "I control my stress." Say it repeatedly until you actually believe what you are saying. Unless you believe it, it means absolutely nothing. Stress is as real as Santa Clause. The only way you can stress about something is if you allow it to have enough weight to be on your mind. Being able to control your thoughts and accepting reality is a duo that is greater than stress. Hear me out. Stress is anything you allow to disrupt your thought process or productivity. Once you allow that thing to disrupt you, it has power over you. Those problems or worries you have are all psychosomatic. The amount of sleep you lose because of a problem is up to you. This, again, is related to knowing that no intangible weight should be able to hold you down. The impact of any issue is up to you. Why? Because stress is not real, and you control your stress.

Subject 1 and Subject 2 are going through similar scenarios. Subject 1 accepts his reality. Subject 2 refuses to accept his reality. Subject 1 has already thought of a way to fix his fuck up. Subject 2 is still trying to overstand how he got here. Subject 1 has already tested his theory. Subject 2 hasn't come up with a plan. Instead he's blaming everyone but himself. Subject 1 is digging himself out of a hole. Subject 1 has also been hit with more bad news. The way he has handled the prior mishap has allowed him to relieve some of the mental burden on himself. Subject 2 receives the same bad news. However, he's spent so much time accepting the responsibility of the first mishap, that this news just adds to his mental weight. Subject 1 has a formula for digging himself out of a dark, mental space. He overstands that he can only control what he can control. Subject 2 believes everything is fixable, but he should not have to fix it. He will forever be dependent on someone else's effort and work. In other words, Subject 2 will always fall victim to stress.

72

There's no point in stressing over shit you can't change. Nothing that mattered yesterday matters today. It cannot be fixed, but it can affect you if you allow it. Stop allowing minimal shit to ruin your day. Nah, fuck that. Stop trying to repair shit you already know is not repairable (especially people). You'll never be able to fix the broken yesterdays, so just build your unbreakable to-morrows. Set your infrastructures to be unbreakable.

I was always taught the more you know your worth, the less like-ly it is to get taken advantage of. The most important key to not stressing is being knowledgeable of your worth and capabilities. We often will let a replaceable person ruin our day(s). No one should be given that power. It's up to you not to give it to them. You might say, "I can't function without him/her," but that's bull-shit. You've been functioning your whole life before him/her just fine. If that person dies, what are you going to do, die too? No. Is it learning the routine of a new person that you fear or the lack of being confident in self enough to open up to a new person? My aunt would always say, "Don't give nuh body ah chance fi dash suttin inna yuh face,"—in other words, don't let anybody think you'll crumble without them. When you know your worth, they'll never assume you can't function without them.

Mental toughness has a lot to do with how much control you give the past. It's disturbing how long we let the negative things affect us and how quickly we let go of fun times. We don't em-brace happiness in the moment. This can be easily taken the wrong way, but the reality is NO ONE GIVES A FUCK. I'm not saying everyone doesn't care, but the majority of people don't. They don't care if you come from a single home, if you're rich, if you were raped, if you're a crack baby, if you're disabled, if you were robbed, if you just lost your child. For example, if you play a competitive sport, the opposing team isn't going to let you win just because you went to a funeral for your mom earlier in the week. They might even say intrusive things about your mom just to throw you off. Once they know they can get a certain reaction from you, you're done.

Depression often consists of self-doubt and the overwhelming feeling of reality. It can also consist of feeling a lack of control; let's be real, everyone wants to be in control. When it comes to depression, your thoughts are the deal breaker. Your thoughts will either make you rich or make you crazy. Stress is the worst thing to allow in your body. Stress does to the mind what crack, coke, pills, and liquor, all together on the same night, does to your body. Stress is like small parasites eating away at your mind. It takes away the pride in your appearance, your judgement, and often, stress impacts your weight because it can change your eating habits. Stress is the devil. That shit will kill you faster than cancer. I had an aunt who had an extreme case of cancer, and I had no clue of it. I'm pretty sure she knew it was cancer, but when the doctors confirmed it, that was like reality punching the wind out of her. You could see drastic changes in her spirit and appearance. It wasn't the cancer that changed her so drastically; it was the stress of knowing she had cancer. I'm not saying to avoid medical diagnosis, but I am suggesting that you don't let what you can't change affect your life to the point where you can't even recognize yourself.

Mental health deals with things that, if not controlled, will cause you to harm yourself. Depression is a big part of mental health for a lot of people, for reasons such as being bullied, a lack of feeling wanted, an overdose of reality and them not being able to deal with it, and a lack of physical movement. In life, the sooner you accept the fact that no excuse is acceptable and nobody cares how rough you had or have it, the sooner you'll be able to sympathize less for yourself. Sympathy is temporary. You will be you forever. There's no escaping that. The best way to deal with this is talk to about it with someone. Even yourself. Always talk about whatever is bothering you to yourself first. Often when going through things, we pity ourselves and always imagine the worst. Then, when we get over it or someone else is going through it, it's like, "Oh wow! I can't believe I was like that."

For me, talking to myself aloud was always the best thing. It helped me to remain accountable for my actions and to play the victim less. It also helped me to realize when I was being unreasonable. The best thing that comes from talking to yourself is that you make less bad decisions. But remember, talk to yourself aloud with questions and answers, causes and effects. But, always let people know you're going through something. Mental health is overlooked to the extent that we don't even realize we have become so susceptible to mental abuse, abandonment, PTSD, and many more ways of living that's not right for any human being. I noticed this when I was in a room full of suburban kids, and murder was the topic. It was so foreign to them.

Unfortunately, by this time in my life, I had already dealt with over 20 deaths of people close to me. One time, I mentioned that someone close to me died; therefore, I wouldn't be around on such-and-such date. They were trying to hug me and shit. My response was, "I don't need any hugs; I'm fine." Now, looking back, I realize that I was comfortable with death. They became mental notes that I learned to live with and put in a pocket, suppressing any emotions attached to the situations. Whether it be lack of love, rape, assault, harassment, bullying, being shot, being incarcerated, etc. talk about it. Accept love, accept attention, accept yourself. Especially for the younger demographic. Kids who were told they have an issue and kids who are wrapped up into the negative way of living—they're all at risk. For the kids who have a following bigger than they are aware of, they are at risk. So, if you're the "big homey" and/or advisor to the youth, tell them the truth.

"AS LONG AS YOUR HEART IS STILL PUMPING, EVERYTHING THAT HAPPENS IS A LESSON."

"This life shit is a marathon, not a race."
– Ermias Asghedom

Casualty vs. Lesson

Splashism: Life is always going to be a fight. It's a war not a battle, a marathon not a sprint. You have time to fix what you've fucked up, if you start now. The only person who has control over your victories and defeats is you. Realistically, they might have been fighting a war, but you might have simply been fighting a battle. The difference is you're a fighter. Everything that has been placed in front of you, you have already defeated. So, this to you is just another battle. On the contrary—the other person—they've never fought a battle, so the smallest thing to them is blown out of proportion and considered war. Often, the privileged or the people who have accomplished the least are the war fighters. Poverty-raised, moral, and principle-driven people are usually the battle fighters. They've been fighting for respect, equality, and acceptance forever. Mentally, you have to be the fighter of the battle not the war. Battles and wars are won mentally, before they are won physically. Once you've mentally decided you can't be fucked with, that will carry you throughout your victories.

As long as your heart is still pumping, everything that happens is a lesson. You become wiser from lessons. You can teach people based on your lessons. Hell, that's what I'm doing as you read each word in this book. Hopefully, with these lessons you never have to take a loss. Hopefully, you die a winner and don't know what a loss feels like from this point on. However, the reality is, we all know what losing feels like, but we don't have to know what a true loss feels like. Losing is in the moment, but a loss has finality. Mentally, you cannot allow someone else to determine if or when you lose. You have the power to fight. On this marathon, keep your feet moving. Put on your favorite pairs of shoes. Kick down every door and side step every roadblock. Sounds cliché, I know. One day, you won't have a mentality of a person who is losing or has loss. Until then, the only Ls we are taking is a lesson. Appreciate that the trying moments will ele-vate you to another level. Trials and tribulations build characte

"When one door is closed, don't you know,
another is open?"
– Robert Marley

Mental Bag Questions:

1. Does what people say about you bother or motivate you?
2. What is the hardest lesson you had to learn? What did it do for you?
3. How often do you try to please people?
4. Which pressures drive you: positive or negative?
5. Do you realize your worth?

_____

_____

_____

_____

_____

_____

_____

_____

_____

_____

_____

_____

_____

_____

_____

_____

_____

_____

_____

"Who put this thing together? Me, that's who!
Who do I trust? Me!" – Tony Montana

Personal Bag

The Personal bag is about perspective, the lens through which we see life and are unapologetically selfish. Overstand the only way you can help people is by first helping yourself. Pouring from an empty glass is impossible. Be cognizant of the fact that all the decisions you make you have to live with. These tools will contribute to the elevation of self and the elimination of toxic friends, choices, and personal lifestyles. You're only going around this thing called life once, so why not do it with people who actually deserve to be around?

Personal Bag Tips:

1. Take advantage of time. Don't waste it.
2. Know your surroundings, and if it isn't for you, change it. If it is stressful or draining, get out of it. If you're the one fucking it up, then fix it, or remove yourself for the sake of the other person.
3. Set goals. What's the point of waking up every day and trying to achieve something if you don't have an end game?
4. Always play devil's advocate with yourself, that way you can potentially see the flaws in your actions. Your shit stinks just as much as everyone else's.
5. Toxic friends are easy to identify once you know yourself.

You have to find stability in your personal life, or at least master the art of staying afloat through the storms. Take a duck for example, calm on the surface but paddling like shit to stay afloat beneath the water. Surround yourself with people who will check you when you make thoughtless decisions. Your friends are supposed to help keep you afloat. If they don't know what goals you have set in life, they will allow you to continuously make thoughtless decisions and self-destruct. The people who actually deserve to be around you will call you out on your bullshit. They will encourage you to be the real you and let go of insecurities. In a way, their job is to be whoever or whatever you need them to be.

While you work on capturing and securing your bags, you're going to lose friends or people you thought were friends. However, part of getting in that bag is motivating your friends to get on top of their shit too, to get in their own bags. Don't ever be foolish enough to believe that your REAL friends will hate you because you changed for the better. I don't care how many nights y'all did careless things together. If they are your real friend, they'll always want better for you. They'll see that your decision to become a better you is working, and they'll do the same. There's a saying in the hood, "real n*ggas link up." It's the same saying as, "Birds of a feather flock together" or "You are who Your friends are." Your Personal bag is only for you to determine.

Are the people you're willing to die for, kill for, risk your freedom for, lose jobs for, disown family for, willing to do the same thing for you? Shit, will they even bring you lunch or get out of bed in the middle of the night for you? You cannot give an arm to people who wouldn't give you a hand. Pay attention to the actions of the people you spend time around and their actions toward you. This will help you determine if they are as equally invested in the friendship as you are. It might not be a "code red" situation, but it'll tell you a lot about their character. An older friend from the neighborhood would always say, "Even when you don't need them, ask them for a favor, and see what type of bullshit they come up with why they can't help you."

Splashism: Be very aware of fake help. Fake help is when people only offer help when they know the help is no longer needed. Example, "If I would've been there for the fight, I would have done such-and-such" or "Damn, you should have told me you were stranded; I would have come to get you" knowing damn well, they wouldn't have done a damn thing. If you don't stay clear of them, they'll have you thinking you can depend on them, and when you finally reach out, you'll be assed out. But you won't be able to blame anyone for that besides yourself. Every situation is your fault to some degree. Even when it's clear you're the victim, you have to hold yourself accountable for allowing someone to get over on you. Not saying to blame yourself, but I am saying hold yourself accountable to avoid the same mishap twice. The isolation required in the Personal bag shall be beneficial in the long run with avoiding being used by people over and over. Not saying everything is your fault; however, as J Cole says, "Fool me one time, shame on you. Fool me twice, can't put the blame on you. Fool me three times, fuck the peace signs. Load the chopper, let it rain on you."

"EXTERNALLY, YOUR BIGGEST WEAKNESS IS THE PEOPLE WE TRUST WHO POSE AS FRIENDS."

"Character consists of what you do on the third and fourth tries."
– James A. Michener

You Quit Too Soon

There are elements you identify as weak and strong that align you to your goal or help you create the construct to your personal pyramid. To expound on that idea, there internal and external strengths and/or weaknesses that prevent success or enhances the likelihood of success. Internally, it could be your resilient attitude, optimism, and aspiration to be great. Externally, it could be your support system, simply people giving you words of encouragement. Weaknesses internally are things such as self-doubt, lack of self-love, hatred, laziness, and anything you allow to rattle you. Externally, your biggest weakness is the people we trust who pose as friends but don't have your best interest at heart. Your surroundings might be your biggest weakness by putting yourself in environments that are not conducive to your well-being. We all need what I call an honest inventory. That's when you really look in the mirror and check yourself, every flaw, and everything about the way you operate. Take all the skeletons out of your closet and dispose of them, face your fears, learn where and how to change to be a better parent, employee, person, friend, caregiver, etc. Forget all the sympathy and excuses that you want to make for yourself. When you check yourself, it's ok to be harsh. The more harsh you are on yourself, the less affected you'll be when someone gives you their opinion of you.

"I HAD TO START BASING MY DECISIONS AROUND WHO WAS QUALIFIED, AND THAT'S WHEN I BEGAN TO NOTICE THE DIFFERENCE."

"Wounds from a sincere friend are better than many kisses from an enemy." – Proverbs 27:6

<u>Ohana</u>

Splashism: Family over everything, right? Bullshit. Before you get all crazy and think I'm telling you that your family doesn't matter or that friends should come before your family, overstand that's not at all what I am implying. Here's my logic: family members are chosen for you. They're inevitable. You have no say so on the family you're born into. But your friends are a real representation of you, and when you make changes, your associates sometimes change also, so they're still a representation of you. Family will sometimes pull that family card at the most strategic and unreasonable times. It's like playing UNO, having one card left and getting hit with a draw four card. Really bro! Family often won't overstand you, and that doesn't mean they don't love you. It's just how things seem to work.

On a daily basis, surround yourself with like-minded individuals. Family or not, don't let that hinder a relationship with a person. I would often guilt trip myself into fucking with someone who is less qualified for whatever situation simply because they were family. I couldn't overstand why I would continuously fall short. That was me being what I call *a victim to loyalty*. Never work solely off of loyalty to a person. More times than none you'll find yourself receiving the short end of the stick. I had to start basing my decisions around who was qualified, and that's when I began to notice the difference. You've got to be a damn fool if you think I'm putting you before people who treat me just as well as I treat them, if not better, simply because we share the same blood—especially in the business world. Don't compromise your safety, finances, or happiness for someone simply because that person is part of your family. Stop letting the word 'FAMILY' be used as reverse psychology to get you to go against your gut feelings or to compromise yourself. I've watched family members steal, kill, and lie on each other, which is what's tainted the meaning for me—not saying friends are any different, but always remember you chose those friends.

How many times have you let your family get away with things your friends could never get away with? How many times have you fucked yourself over for your family? Do you regret it?

_____
_____
_____
_____
_____
_____
_____
_____
_____
_____
_____
_____
_____
_____
_____
_____
_____
_____
_____
_____
_____
_____
_____
_____
_____

"It is mental slavery to cling to things that have stopped serving their purpose in your life."
– Chinonye J. Chidolue

The 9 to 5 Program

Splashism: 9-to-5ing yourself is when you force yourself to do something you don't want to do but feel like you should. Let's be honest: nobody wants a 9 to 5, but everyone has them because you have to get by. Even in relationships, people often stay when they don't want to because they don't know how to be alone or because they don't want to hurt someone by leaving. What if you're hurting yourself by staying? That's 9-to-5ing yourself. You're limiting your reach. A 9-to-5 is eight hours during which you do what you're told, when you're told, and how you're told. There is no reaching for the stars, no dreaming, and no taking risks. There are just tasks set by 'management,' so your ceiling isn't as high as the dreamers. You've been put into a box.

When you're in a situation and you feel as if you're trapped, you must learn that—yes, it might be where you want to be, but it isn't where you need or have to be. Yes, that person might have the best interest for you, but don't 9-to-5 yourself. Don't allow others to put you in a box. Don't put yourself in a box. Boxing yourself in limits your reach, your optimism, and your greatness. It limits you from using the tools you were born with and sprinkling tools you have learned from others. In any partnership, things run their course.

So yes, your job may pay well, but are you draining yourself mentally and spiritually every time you go to work? The bag theory is about overstanding your worth and your value and not minimizing the expectations you have of yourself.

List ways that you're 9-to-5ing yourself:

_____

_____

_____

_____

_____

_____

_____

_____

_____

_____

_____

_____

_____

_____

_____

_____

_____

_____

_____

_____

_____

_____

_____

_____

_____

_____

_____

_____

"Do nothing out of selfish ambition or vain conceit. Rather, in humility value others above yourselves."
– Philippians 2:3

Pride

When's the last time you made a good decision based on pride? I'm willing to bet you can't name more than three. Pride is a gift and a curse. You have to learn to swallow your pride and to accept humility. Growing up, I was taught people should "die for their pride." This is the biggest battle I face to this day; you have to counter the urge of letting your pride get in the way by simply reminding yourself that some things just aren't worth getting the best of you.

Think of all the decisions you've made based solely on pride. How many of those decisions were any good? After this paragraph, you can write down all the good and bad decisions that were made because of pride to help you realize how many of your bad decisions were made out of pride. Most of my friends who are locked up for putting in work felt like, "a nigga tried to play them," and they weren't going for it. Imagine how much they regret their decision now. I talk to some of my old heads, and they always say the same thing: "Let that pride shit go." Don't belittle yourself or allow yourself to be taken advantage of, but when you feel your pride has been violated, think before you retaliate. I'm not telling you not to be prideful because there are good kinds of pride, but know when to act on your pride and emotion and when not to act on it. Pride is only good when logical thinking and actions stem from it.

Name three decisions you made solely based on pride?

_____
_____
_____
_____
_____
_____
_____
_____
_____
_____
_____
_____
_____
_____
_____
_____
_____
_____
_____
_____
_____
_____
_____
_____
_____
_____
_____
_____
_____

The lines above will probably be your most filled in section.
That's okay. That was the point. Pride is a muthafucker!
LET. IT. GO!

"I'm just a product of my environment, and it comes out in the music." – Antwan André Patton

<u>The Shmurdas</u>

<u>*Splashism*</u>: Imagine being two young kids from one of the most known cities in the world and performing your hit song at a sold-out show in your hometown. Those kids were Bobby Shmurda and Rowdy Rebel, two of the biggest rappers in recent years. They made an impression for crimes they allegedly committed and then rapped about. Bobby Shmurda, in an interview said he had an opportunity to do even less time than he was initially given, but his loyalty to his friend, Rowdy, was too strong.

Shmurda replied, "I did it for Rowdy. They offered me five and offered Rowdy twelve. They said the only way they'll give him seven is if I took seven, too. So, you know, I had to take one for the dawg."[6]

Bobby also explained the injustice of the situation. "The judge wasn't really playing fair because he was letting a lot of stuff into court that wasn't supposed to be. The only witnesses the DA had against us were lying cops. We had detectives lying, saying they seen us with guns in our hands, but when everything came back there was no DNA, no fingerprints, no nothing. My lawyer told me we don't want to go to court in Manhattan with these white people because they're going to be looking at me, a little Black kid, suspiciously. Who are they going to believe: the word of this Black kid talking about shooting shit up or the words of White officers? A jury is going to believe cops all day. We're Black kids; these are White people with badges."[6]

We can all learn something about loyalty. Loyalty: nobody owes you that shit, and you owe it to no one! Make sure you can live with your choices though, when it comes to who you are loyal to. You know the saying, "You do the crime, you do the time"? Those are the rules for the everyday civilians. In the streets, "If you get caught, you do the time." Again, that's a choice you have

---

6   (Diaz 2016)

to make. Can you live with yourself knowing you ratted someone out? Can you live with yourself knowing you didn't snitch when you get hit with 15 years or more and your co-defendant is at home acting like you never existed? Are you going to wish you snitched? That's something you have to answer for yourself.

Bobby was willing to sacrifice 2.5 years of his life in order to eliminate 5 years of his "dawg's" sentence. This kind of loyalty is not only about the Personal bag, this is about the Spiritual bag as well. He knew deep down that had he not taken the 7 years, he wouldn't have been able to stomach his own reflection in the mirror. The Spiritual bag is about being happy with yourself and your decisions. Remember, earlier we talked about giving an arm for people who wouldn't give a hand to you? In the case of Bobby and Rowdy, they were two people who stood up for each other. They could have easily snitched and lied on one another. Bobby knew Rowdy was going to 'stand up' and take the best offer instead of telling because he trusted and overstood him. By stand up, I mean metaphorically—accepting the consequences of your actions without tucking your tail. This is why knowing your circle is so critical. Have people around you who you can see yourself in. Bobby played by the rules of the gang, which is, "LOYALTY comes first." Loyalty is a major component to his life.

A part of the Personal bag is the image you choose to represent you. Bobby pointed out that he couldn't trust his image (Mugshot Theory) in court with that jury. He stated, "They weren't going to believe the words of a Black kid who talked about shooting shit up." Remember, whatever you say, do, or post will and can be used against you. Not just in the court of law but in the 'court of life.' You have to be aware of the way you represent yourself. Bobby and Rowdy were two kids in their early 20s who made songs that completely changed their lives for what seemed like the better. These songs could've simply been about the life of people around them in their neighborhood or what they see on social media, but since those songs came out of their mouths, the content of the songs is attached to them. Imagine getting ready to fight a case where they don't have much evidence, but because there is a video of you rapping lyrics that may or may not be about your life, those videos are used against you to bury you under the jail.

Let's look at this idea of image in a more general way. Not

maintaining or protecting your image is like tweeting offensive rap lyrics and then getting offended when people associate you with the content of those lyrics at a job interview. Or rappers who talk "shoot'em up, bang bang" in their rap disses, then play victim when the opposition approaches them with that energy and they want to cry wolf. You have the chance to steer people to the perception you want them to have of you. One thing you can somewhat control is someone's mind when it comes to a perception of you.

No, this part of the book is not to glorify thugs, violence, or doing jail time. It's to show that regardless of the circumstances, no one can take any of your bags. This is confirmation that only you can take your bags from you. Having a troubled past doesn't mean you can't capture your bags moving forward. Your past doesn't matter, it doesn't have to dictate your future unless you allow it

The 5 Tools of the Shmurdas

1. Know your friends, and be able to read their energy. Be able to realize their actions are transparent, but the situations aren't. So, when they complain about something small just know in a more severe situation, they'll complain even more.
2. No matter the situation, never go against your code. You have to be able to look at you in the mirror for the rest of your life.
3. Loyalty trumps love and money! I'm sure he loves his mother and family and wishes he could get back to them, but the loyalty to himself and what he believes in overrules all.
4. Whatever image you portray is what people remember. Whether you're really like that or not!
5. Most importantly, NEVER go against the code; it makes it so much easier for you to live with yourself

"I don't care what you think you saw. The fuck is you gone believe: me or your eyes?"
– Maurice Eastwood

Mugshot Theory

Splashism: A mugshot is the photo police take of people after they've been caught or accused of doing something and taken into custody for it. Once your mugshot surfaces, your reputation is tarnished. Unfortunately, every accomplishment you've achieved is somewhat tainted. By this time, everyone's true opinion of you is publicly revealed: loved-ones, co-workers, strangers, enemies, everyone. It's like they forget a mugshot DOES NOT mean you are guilty. Maybe people should smile more in their mugshot photo. With mugshots come perception.

When a person's mugshot is released, a picture gets painted of that person by everyone. A picture says a thousand words, but you never know what those thousand words can be. Sometimes, those words are bullshit. When you present yourself to the public, always consider your first impression and daily impression as your mugshot. The words you use and your actions are what/ who you're being accused of being. People will judge all you've done, good or bad, based on what they remember you for.

Your social media is also your mugshot, especially for people you don't personally know. If you're flashing guns, they'll call you a thug (if you're Black), and that's on you for being on the Internet actin' like you "bout that life." If all you share are pictures of your body and sexual memes but get mad someone makes a sexual comment, you can only blame yourself. Not because it gives them a right to comment but because you're supposed to be smart enough to know how shallow and simple-minded the world is. We take the blame even when it's not our fault, so that we can be quicker and more advanced than the competition. Social media mugshots are powerful because they're often the only image the world sees, and you can basically kiss your real identity goodbye. Motherfuckas don't care about the truth. Remember, there's two sides to you. If someone knows you one way due to your mugshot, when they see you, they'll always

95

think of you like that. For example, let's say you know James from selling weed and being a street dude, then you see him making a presentation to your college class, introducing his invention. Now imagine the opposite: meeting him during a presentation, then finding out he's your local Pablo Escobar. Your idea of James wouldn't be the same at all. Your first impression is everlasting.

"IT'S LIKE THEY FORGET A MUGSHOT DOES NOT MEAN YOU ARE GUILTY."

"I keep my head high, I got my wings to carry me. I don't know freedom, I want my dreams to rescue me."
– Jermaine Cole

Opportunity To Be The Opportunity

Don't cost yourself a great opportunity because you aren't ready. Preparation is critical. As they say, "Practice makes perfect" or "stay ready, so you ain't gotta get ready." Missing out on opportunities will eventually result in you missing out on being the opportunity. What I mean by this is, not being prepared for any opportunity can cost you an opportunity to make a difference for the people around you and yourself. You must try to capitalize on any opportunity presented to you that has a positive outcome.

I was born in a developing country, so anything I get is an opportunity. That's my motivation. I tell myself that, and I believe that had my family not migrated to this country, my options would have been limited due to my environment. I emphasize on making the most out of the privilege my family provided. A lot of people say America isn't the land of opportunity, but shit, we get to go to school for free in America. That's an opportunity compared to where I come from. You have to overstand the value you possess, the position you are in, and the privileges you overlook on a daily basis. I'm sure Steve Jobs didn't know he would be able to provide so much employment, but he seized on the opportunities before him and turned them into opportunities for others. Lebron James' work ethic put him in the position to be able to take advantage of every opportunity in front of him, and now he can provide jobs for his friends and others for generations. It's imperative to use the benefits of being successful to help push everyone forward.

Be the opportunity for those who come after you. You will be the beginning of a whole generation. Yes, you'll have children if you're lucky enough, and they'll have children and so on. The power plays you make now can be the difference in what they experience. So, before you sell certain shit or fail to capitalize on something, think about the difference you can make—not just for you but for the legacy you will leave behind. Get out of the mindset of thinking small. This book ain't for smallminded people. When you have a few extra dollars, don't go buy designer. Don't go to the bar. Save it, buy a book, do something that'll add value and substance. Learn how to capitalize and become the superior you that you aspire to be.

"BE THE OPPOR-TUNITY FOR THOSE WHO COME AFTER YOU."

"Deserve your dream." – Octavio Paz

You Don't Deserve Shit

You have to look for opportunities. People will always tell you to pray for it and to speak it into existence. I'm telling you to get up off your ass, make a way out of no way, and get to it. I've seen my mom make a way out of no way. I've seen my grandma make a way out of no way. I've seen my homey be in the hole 10, 20, 30...100 grand and get back. I'm sure you've experienced failing a class and found a way out with a passing grade, not because you felt you deserved it but because you wanted it. YOU DON'T DESERVE SHIT IN LIFE.

Continuously saying what you think you deserve won't make things go your way. You don't deserve shit, but you do need to know what you want! Strive for what you want, not what you believe you deserve. There is no such thing as wanting too much when you're the one providing it. Ain't no such thing as too much love for self or too much ambition or too much of anything you're doing for you. As humans, we can only absorb so much in a day. The Personal bag is about being selfish. Dodging the energy vultures and catering to self. If there are 365 days in the year, and you want to have 365 pairs of socks then shit, if you can afford'em, buy'em. It's only too much when it's coming from someone else because they can limit what they want to give. If you're a person who is always helping and has a hard time saying "NO," then why would you want what you deserve as opposed to what you want? I want enough to help everyone else and still be able to do my damn thing without checking my account balance or telling myself I'll just get it next week. Don't you want enough food to feed everyone and still have food? Don't you want enough space in your house that you don't have to hear the kids in the other room? Well, bust your ass for it because you want it. Believing you deserve something or are owed something will only help you build excuses when you don't get that thing. Evaluate what you're doing and whether it's enough to have the high expectations you have. Are you giving what you want your all?

99

Write down your wants and what you believe you deserve in relationships, at work, financially, and just our overall life:

_____

_____

_____

_____

_____

_____

_____

_____

_____

_____

_____

_____

_____

_____

_____

_____

_____

_____

_____

_____

_____

_____

_____

_____

_____

Personal Bag Questions

1. How often do you make decisions that are best for some-one else?
2. When's the last time you said, "Fuck everybody" and did something for you?
3. Do you know when it is time for you to change your per-sonal surroundings? Do you have a strategy to change your personal surroundings?
4. Do you know how to separate business from pleasure?
5. Can you handle all the success you ask for?

*"A plant-based diet kinda makes your soul lighter.
I had a newfound respect for all life."*
– David Styles

Health Bag

The tools inside of the Health bag will assist you in taking notice of what you attempt to fuel your body with and how you treat your body. Hopefully, with these tools, you'll eventually treat your body better than any material object you own. Overstanding that sleep, food intake, physical activity, and the daily consumption of water will help reduce many health risks. The body is a temple and should be treated as such.

Health Bag Tips:
1. Drink water.
2. Monitor what and when you eat.
3. Sleep. You're not 7-years-old—staying up all night isn't 'cool." It's foolish.
4. Get tested.
5. TAKE CARE OF YOUR DAMN HYGIENE!

The first thing you should do when capturing the Health bag is conduct an internal scan of self and be knowledgeable enough to know it doesn't have to feel like something is wrong for something to be wrong. Know that what you eat and drink is possibly damaging you slowly. Become one with your body, take the time to read labels, books, and to watch videos on health. You only get one life and one body. Take care of that shit. Getting in the Health bag is continuous. It's fighting the urge of that Little Debbie snack, the salt, or those GMO filled wings from your favorite spot; it's pissing after sex to avoid a UTI, drinking less of that poisonous ass Hennessy and Patron, which is killing your liver. Detox, especially if your body is consuming drugs and alcohol on a weekly basis.

Splashism: What are you fueling your body with? Nutrition is a chain reaction: you are what you eat. Think of it like gas for your car. If you're driving a heavy-duty truck or a foreign car, why would you fuel yourself with 87 Unleaded gas when 93 Premium exists? Think of your body as your dream car. I say dream car because whenever I put 93 in my Honda Accord, my friends say I act as if my Honda is a Lamborghini. I just reply, "If I treat it like a million-dollar car, it'll last me forever." Same with your body. If you're out of shape and trying to get in shape, no matter who you are, your dream body/car will always need 93 Premium gas. The other fuels/food might be cheaper, but they aren't better. In most areas of life, it is rare that cheaper is better. Cheaper food might taste better to you because it's what you're used to, but what it does to your insides long term isn't worth the money you'll save by consistently taking the cheap route. If your body is a foreign car or even a big boy pick-up truck, you must fuel it as such. Don't treat yourself like a piece of shit car.

87/Regular	_89/Mid-grade_	_93/Premium_
Pastries/ Cookies/Cakes	Peanut Butter	Organic/Free Range Chicken or no meat at all
Arizona Tea/ Big Burst/Soda	Egg Yolk	Non-GMO Organic Fruits
Pizza	Bananas	Fresh Green Vegetables
White Bread	Cold Cuts	Water/Natural Juices
Processed Juices	Cow's Milk	Salmon
French Fries/ Potato Chips	Potatoes	Almond/ Cashew Milk
Ice Cream	Canned Tuna	Raw Nuts
Most Fast Food Restaurants	Beef	Egg Whites
Processed Meat/Food	Rice	Sweet Potatoes

If you really give it thought, there's rarely anything in life that you can buy where the cheaper version is better for you. So, why in the hell do you think that cheaper foods are better for you? I'm going to say this one last time: your body is a fucking temple. A temple is a dwelling place of a God or Gods. So, treat it as such! Care for it. Pay attention to it. Nurture it.

The reality is, a lot of people live in poverty. They struggle to afford healthier and more costly foods. It would be extremely brash of me to just say buy expensive food because you have to. If you can't afford it, instead of eating less or more expensive things just change what you eat and how much of it you eat. For example, pay attention to serving sizes. **Pay attention to the amount of sugar you put in your body.** No matter what you do, do not go a day without drinking water!

"PAY ATTENTION TO THE AMOUNT OF SUGAR YOU PUT IN YOUR BODY."

"Living life is a choice. Making a difference in someone else's isn't." – Scott Mescudi

The 5 Benefits of Drinking Water:

1. **Water flushes bodily waste** – drink water to get the bullshit you've been putting in your body out of your body.
2. **It helps to maintain blood pressure** – the less water you drink, the more likely your blood will become thicker, which will increase your blood pressure.
3. *It makes minerals and nutrients accessible* – for minerals and nutrients to reach the necessary destinations in your body, water assists them in getting where they belong.
4. **It delivers oxygen throughout the body** – adult humans are 60 percent water, and our blood is 90 percent water; blood carries oxygen to different parts of the body.
5. **Weight Loss** – water may also help with weight loss, if it is consumed instead of sweetened juices and sodas. "Preloading" with water before meals can also help prevent overeating by creating a sense of fullness.

List 5 things you'll eliminate from your diet:

1. _____
2. _____
3. _____
4. _____
5. _____

When you are fully dedicated and motivated, you can intentionally track your food intake by making charts based on what exactly you're trying to do health wise: gain and tone muscle, lose fat, or whatever the case may be. Challenge yourself to see if your body can keep up with your mind and vice versa. In order for your body to do what your mind wants it to do, you have to both fuel and push yourself every day. However, you can't stop there. Your thoughts won't be right if you're allowing negativity inside of your mind and body. There has to be teamwork between your mind and body. They have to be parallel to each other. Mentally, you have to be able to look at the worst situation and tell yourself you can get through it. Physically, you have to be fueled the right way to withstand the challenges and physical strain adversity will put on your body. Mentally, you have to look at hurdles and be spearheaded enough to know YOU WILL NOT BE DEFEATED.

In addition to keeping your body toned and healthy, regular physical activity can help keep your thinking, learning, and judgment skills on point as you get older. It can also reduce your risk of depression and may help you sleep better. Studies have shown that doing aerobics or a mix of aerobics and muscle-strengthening activities 3 to 5 times a week for 30 to 60 minutes can give you these health benefits. Some scientific evidence has also shown that even lower intensity physical activity can be beneficial.

You may not have time to go to the gym. You may not have the money to be a member of a gym. You may not have a babysitter while you're at the gym. None of that has to stop you from getting the basic level of physical activity at home. There are a bunch of workouts you can do from home that'll have optimal results, as long as you do them correctly and frequently. You don't need much space or equipment to do ab workouts, wall sits, speed squats, planks, toe raises, push-ups, or even stretches. Doing some of these exercises 10-25 times each commercial break on a daily basis will be beneficial to your body and health goals. You can even do this while traveling. On a road trip, every time you stop for gas, food, to use the bathroom, and/or to rest, you can do squats and push-ups. However or wherever you work out, you have to go hard.

"ANY PHYSICAL ACTIVITY DONE WHILE IN THE SUN FLUSHES THE BODY OF ANYTHING TOXIC."

Examples of cardio that don't require a gym membership:

1. Jumping Jacks
2. Jump Rope
3. Jogs
4. Push Up
5. Sit-Ups
6. Walking
7. Bike riding
8. Swimming
9. Yoga
10. Squatting

I never realized the importance and the peace of mind a good diet and great exercise brings you. Personally, being physically active on a consistent basis unlocks the ability to maintain clearer thoughts and eliminates having a sluggish feeling body. I'm not sure of the science behind this, but the shit is amazing. When it's nice outside, spend some time partaking in activities in the sun. Any physical activity done while in the sun flushes the body of anything toxic. I'm not a doctor or a scientist but luckily, you don't need to be when you have Google and a little bit of brains. I looked up the good the sun does for you, and one thing that stood out to me was that the sun plays such an intricate part in how Vitamin D fuels your body. There have been studies that show depression occurs in people during the change of seasons. As winter approaches and the earth tilts away from the sun, the days become shorter. This means less sunlight is available for our use. Many people find themselves depressed at this time of year, and the cause has been linked to the lack of sunlight. Indeed, people who sit under lamps that recreate the light spectrum of the sun have reported feeling happier and more energized. Sunlight also stimulates the pineal gland deep in the brain. In other words, take your ass outside! Take in some sun. It'll boost your energy as a person to contribute to your happiness.

"Extreme poverty anywhere is a threat to human security everywhere." — Kofi Annan

Food Deserts

Splashism: Eating McDonalds, Wendys, and Burger King on the daily isn't doing anything for you except filling up your stomach. Fried foods aren't the best choice either. I'm a firm believer that you get what you pay for, so when you're drinking Arizona and Brisk tea, Hawaiian Punch, and Big Bursts, just know it's not benefiting you in any way. I am not telling you what to eat, but if your whole family has high blood pressure or suffers from Diabetes, then the baglike thing to do would be to monitor your diet. Stay away from cheap ass juices and sodas, and take it easy on the greasy foods. Also, don't overcook your food; it can lead to the formation of harmful compounds that raise the risk of cancer. Leading cancer foods include canned food, GMO foods, red meat, refined sugar, sugary drinks, salty foods, white bread, farmed fish, alcohol, microwave popcorn. Unfortunately, the reality is some of the shit they feed us in the inner city is packaged and fed to us to basically wipe us out one way or another.

With the setup of food deserts, it's practically impossible for some people to eat anything good for them. A food desert is an area, often one with poverty-stricken residents, that has little to no access to affordable and nutritious foods (natural foods). As opposed to a food oasis, which is an area with easy access to supermarkets or vegetable shops. In other words, the ghetto is a food desert by design. They feed us shit that pumps estrogen into our bodies, hormone-infested meat, alcohol, and fast food options on every corner or every quarter mile. But there's no grocery stores in the inner city that sell natural foods. It's pretty unfortunate that we can't find natural fruit. Shit, it's pretty fucked up there is even a such thing as fake foods. Geographically speaking, as I sit here and write this book, I am able to name 11 different liquor stores and 24 corner stores all within a one mile radius of where I live. In order for me to find a large chain grocery store with organic foods, I would have to drive 15 minutes or 3.8 miles from my home.

I'll never forget the day I was eating an orange and realized there weren't any seeds. I began to wonder, *how the fuck is this supposed to be a natural fruit with no seeds.* I said to myself, "Maybe I should eat another, that's probably where all the seeds are." After eight oranges and not one seed found, I sat there for a while wondering, *did I just poison myself by eating fake fruits?* "No way these shits are NATURAL without any seeds. How did oranges get planted, grow on a tree, and then have no seeds. This shit is fake as hell. Why the hell are they selling fake fruit." I went on a rant for about an hour at home, and everyone ignored me. Finally, I got the attention of my aunt, but all she said was that I'm crazy and, "The orange is sweet and good to me." Like most people, all she cared about was that it tasted good—not what it was doing to them. Moral of the story is: be aware of what it is that you're eating. Google is accessible. Look it up.

I read a book titled, How to Hustle and Win,[7] and it talked about how pigs were being used as street sweepers, before we had actual street sweepers. It is said when the roads were extremely dirty, they'd load up several pigs into the truck and bring them to the area that needed to be clean. The pigs would walk around, and eat up all the trash. Other animals might sniff around the trash, but pigs would literally eat up all the garbage. I'm sure the pig's owner had no worries because they'd still eat that pig or sell it to be eaten. I wondered if they would get sick or die from the trash. As I read the book, it also mentioned pigs can't be poisoned. They don't have pores, so they roll around in their own waste (shit) to cool down. Also, they only have one stomach, so it's harder for toxic things to exit their body.

In the book, the author says, "Ask people why they eat pork, knowing it's the worst thing you could put in your body, I bet they'll say because it tastes good. He then says, "Ask them, if shit tastes good, would you eat that too?" Ha-ha! I mean, that's a bit excessive, but basically what he's saying is, "If your only reason for eating something, knowing the health difficulties that come with it, is because it tastes good, the likelihood is that you probably shouldn't be eating it. It reminds me of when I was a kid; some of my family didn't eat meat or dairy, some didn't eat pork, and some ate everything except pork. I always wondered what the confusion was as far as why everyone didn't eat the

---

7   (Understanding 2010)

same thing. My uncle would show me VHS videos about the killing of animals and how they made fake meats, etc. Yet, I'd still order that 6-piece nugget. Not because I didn't believe the video but because it tasted good. Now that I am older, I'm not the healthiest person, but I am a lot more conscious of how I eat more so than what I eat. We need to stop eating like we do not love ourselves, when we have an option to eat better. Certain things minorities eat come from the scraps enslaved people were forced to eat. For instance, neck bones, hog head cheese, pig's feet—those were scraps. That shit ain't healthy. Again, I'm not telling you what to eat, but what I am telling you is to monitor how much of it you consume. When it comes to animals, if you have the plant based option for any type of meat that's the better choice to make. So, if you want to eat pork, beef, and/or chicken, the least you could do is go the free range, non-GMO, plant-based route. Give yourself a chance of longevity; there's already enough things killing us. For you people who shun others for eating animals but still drink alcohol, that shit does the same damage if not worse. Cigarettes and alcohol fuck up the body just as well as these bullshit chicken nugget meals we eat.

I'm not gone bullshit like it's not a known thing that vegan life is the healthiest way to go. It isn't easy or cheap, but we have to find a way to get as close to clean eating as possible! As much time as you spend gossiping, you should spend asking family members how often they check their blood pressure, encouraging them to drink water, calling them up to go for a walk/jog— anything. Be proactive. If you come from a family with a history of Diabetes, simple things will help you like diluting your drinks and putting less salt in food. If your family members aren't getting regular check-ups, ask them why. Too often I hear people say, "I just don't feel like going today," "I don't want to know what's wrong with me" or "I'll make an appointment when I get some free time." Turn up a little less. Take care of your body a lot more. Sleep more. If you can afford to eat better, do so. If eating good was easy and/or cheap more people would do it. It's not easy, but it is doable.

"CIGARETTES AND ALCOHOL FUCK UP THE BODY JUST AS WELL AS THESE BULLSHIT CHICKEN NUGGET MEALS WE EAT."

"Lighten up on yourself. No one is perfect.
Gently accept your humanness."
– Deborah Day

Talk About Doing The Do!

It would be unbaglike of me to talk about health and not write about sex. When referring to health, people only think about physical fitness, nutrition, and whether your body has experienced any broken bones, surgeries, irregularities, or illnesses. Sexual intercourse should always be talked about during conversations about health, even if the only advice you have to give is to "wrap it up." Often, I hear people say, "Everybody is really having sex with everybody," yet that same person will still have unprotected sex and be confused when they get a sexually transmitted disease. How are you so sure the person you're having sex with is only having sex with you, especially if he/she isn't the only person you're having sex with? I'm always hearing statements like, "Yo, that shit feel so good without a condom," but does it feel good enough to have a baby? How about to catch an STD? When you ask that it becomes an entirely different conversation filled with delusional beliefs that it won't happen to them. Things happen and sometimes you just aren't prepared, but if you stay ready you don't have to get ready. I'm not saying not to have sex, but I am saying be responsible and realistic as to how and why you're in the situations you're in. Keeping condoms is essential for men and women who are having casual sex. Get regular checkups, and always communicate with your partner(s). Don't be the selfish fuck who thinks they have something and doesn't check on it.

A CONDOM IS CHEAPER THAN:

- BABY WIPES
- DIAPERS
- ENFAMIL
- BABY BOTTLES
- BABY CLOTHES
- EVERYTHING BABY RELATED

"I can stop if I really want to." – every addict ever

Is it Worth The Fun?

Have you ever seen a real-life alcoholic? If so, I'm sure you've noticed how bad they smell. I'm also sure you're aware of the changes in their actions, like the outrageous shit they say, the erratic behavior, and their unpredictability. Sometimes, it's the things people go through that they can't handle. Sometimes, it's simply people not taking advantage of what they control and then losing a grip on life. In which case, addiction of any sort is a coping mechanism that they can't shake. Pill addiction is the tricky one; some people I know were on pain meds after a car accident or after being shot, and some people I know started popping pills to experience fun and got hooked. Both always say the same thing, "How hard it is to stop taking them?" Then when you try to talk them out of it, the main thing they say as a response is, "Chill. it's not coke or crack; it's not heroin or dope. It's just pills." You ever seen a real coke head? Even Bobby Brown didn't make music about coke, but you damn sure could tell he was on it. The people around him noticed his behavior before he noticed they noticed. Basically, what I am trying to say is others will realize your behavior is off before you will, and it will cause conflict and confusion in whatever relationship you guys have because you're unable to control yourself.

The more you drink promethazine codeine, the more dependent you'll become! *"Lean gives you such stomach pain. I'll never forget the time I was at South by Southwest and had to do all these shows, and I was sitting on the couch curled up, hours of pain. That wasn't the moment I quit, that was the moment I said I need more,"* said Schoolboy Q in an interview. In reality, your body has now become used to these drugs, and instead of cutting back, you feed yourself more to avoid the pain you'd experience during withdrawal. You also might remember when Gucci Mane was going on his Twitter rant and seemed to be making up a bunch of fabricated stories? That was largely due to his lean consumption. *"I've been drinking lean for 10 plus years, and I must admit it has destroyed me. I want to be the first rapper to admit I'm addicted to lean and that shit ain't no joke,"* he continued. *"I can barely*

(115)

remember all the things I've done and said. However, there's no excuse." [8]

It appears people no longer know how to be sober. From weed to pills to alcohol, people seem to be enslaved. However, health is the state of being free from illness or injury, whether that illness or injury is internal or external, whether it be in the body or in the brain.

There's always a huge discussion about whether or not weed is really considered a drug. Personally speaking, I've seen weed be the demise of some of my friends. I'm not completely against weed, but for some people, it triggers certain chemical imbalances. I've seen a bad batch of weed ruin people's life for good. If you know a lot of your family members or friends got their weed "laced" at some point, then why are you smoking with them. If you know they smoke dust, and all this other type of weed, why smoke with them? If they're a stranger, then why are you smoking with them? If you weren't there when the spliff was being rolled, then why are you smoking with them? All I'm suggesting is, if you're going to smoke weed, be cautious and know what you're putting into your body. Be cautious, and be smart. Also, if all you do is smoke and drink, clearly you need a break to detox your body and remove some of the waste and poison you're filling your body with. You should also accept that you have an addiction, and try to control it. Remember, if you do drugs, don't let them do you. Meaning, do not become a slave to your drug of choice.

There's enough man-made shit put on this world to destroy us internally and externally, so what I am asking is that you give yourself a chance. Do not self-destruct. Don't taint your body. Be mindful. Be loving. Be proactive. Remember, you only get to do this life shit once.

"EVERYBODY IS REALLY HAVING SEX WITH EVERYBODY."

8   (Twitter 2013) (Understanding 2010) (Understanding 2010)

1. Why continuously do and consume things that are clearly damaging your body?
2. How are you going to implement exercise into your schedule?
3. What will you substitute from your daily diet from the food grade chart?
4. What is the main thing you want to improve about yourself physically?
5. How often do you go to the doctor?

_____
_____
_____
_____
_____
_____
_____
_____
_____
_____
_____
_____
_____
_____
_____
_____
_____
_____
_____
_____

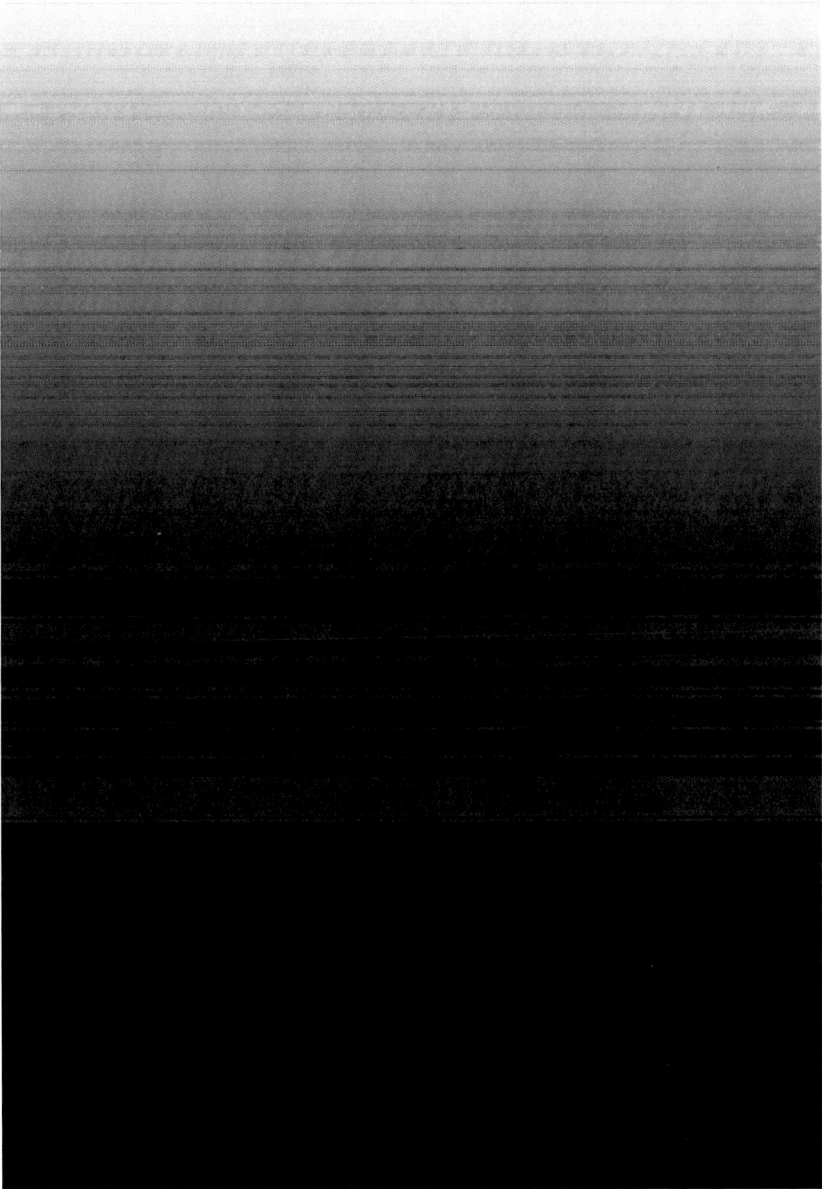

"Sometimes our dreams come true,
sometimes our fears do too."
– Jermaine Cole

Financial Bag

The last of the tools is the Financial bag. These tools will help you prioritize your lifestyle to be financially equipped to do whatever it is that you aspire. These tools will force you to take heed of your priorities. The financial bag aspires to add motivation and attention to detail and encourages you to think of your financial track history going forward as your legacy. No amount of money will ever make you whole, so never lose your morals for it.

Financial Bag Tips:

1. Get a whiteboard and plot. Visualize your plans and write them down. A plan is better when you can see it.
2. Invest in your goals.
3. Plan your strategy before you execute your plan.
4. Don't buy one if you can't afford two.
5. Never compromise your integrity for any dollar amount.

"STOP SAYING YOU'RE BROKE; THAT'S A MINDSET. JUST SAY YOUR MONEY IS ON HOLD."

"Money is numbers, and numbers never end. If it takes money to be happy, your search for happiness will never end."
– Robert Marley

The 5<u>th</u> Bag

I put the Financial bag last in this book because I feel like, in the game of life, money will be the least of your worries once you've captured, secured, and gotten in the other four bags. Making money is similar to a sport game; any athlete can attest to the fact that when you are giving it all your effort, things just go your way. There's no set formula to doing things the right way, but once you've figured out what formulas have worked for you and helped you capture the other four bags, you will have your framework for securing your Financial bag.

If your loyalty, love, or genuineness depends on how much money you have, then you have a lot of reevaluating to do. You should probably revisit one of the first three bags. My grand-mother used to always tell me, "Stop saying you're broke; that's a mindset. Just say your money is on hold." I used to wonder what she meant, but what she was telling me was that saying you're broke is not something you should put into the universe because it might actually become who you think you are. She'd also tell me, "Don't do it for the money; that will come. You have to love what you are doing and believe in it." It's obvious when you're doing something out of love as opposed to doing it for money or acceptance. When you do it for money, something is going to backfire, and when it does, you'll crack because it was never real for you. You won't know how to fix it and get it right.

Let the securing of the other four bags be your infrastructure for capturing the Financial bag. The steps taken for those bags will help bring financial opportunities for you to dominate because you've been building yourself to be prepared for these opportuni-ties to present themselves. Living by certain morals, values, and principles will fill the emptiness you think acceptance of others will give you if you have money. Honestly, if these people only want to be around because you have money, what do you think will happen when the money goes?

"Never fall out over no money or how pretty she is."
– Kadeem Jackson

The $40,000 Lesson

"Today is November 21, 2017, and I have $3 cash in my pocket and $300 in the bank. Yesterday I had $40,303.00 to my name. I made a bad decision and moved too fast, and it caused me to lose it all at once, resulting in one of the hardest financial lessons ever. Now I'm down on my ass financially. All the financial goals I wanted to reach were no longer possible, at least at the moment. I'm not sure what my next move is. I just know it has to be my best move yet. A lesson like this is traumatizing. I ain't got no emotions, no mood, and my thought process is everywhere. I mean, I could hit a lick...hit a lick, steal, see if it's lit in the field. Those are the easiest ways to make a little change. Now I have the pressure of being watched. I'm paranoid, feeling like I want to throw up even though I haven't eaten. Fortunately, my friends ain't babying me. They told me I fucked up, then followed up by saying things like, "It's just money. It could be worse," and "At least you have your freedom." The realest shit said was, "I thought you were the enTRAPreneur; bounce back, you God in the flesh, right?" I remember sitting up and saying to myself, "Stop bitching about it, and take accountability. I am an enTRA-Preneur, and if I had any doubts, now is the time to show up and prove myself to myself. How can I want people who have nothing to believe in my system, if I'm crying over $40,000.00?"
– my journal

"IT'S VERY RARE THAT MONEY BRINGS YOU JOY."

"I want the finer things in my life, so I hustle."
– Curtis Jackson

For the Love of the Green

Why is it that money costs so much? It costs the time you spend trying to make money, and the amount of time spent making it is not even remotely close to how quickly the money goes. It costs the pain you feel when you make sacrifices for the money, the pressure you feel when everyone and everything needs or costs money, the blood that is spilled in pursuit of money, the family going hours unattended to make the money, sweat and tears that drip as you grind for the money. Too often I see people going to jail and they can't even cover their ass with a good lawyer, but they have thousands of dollars of material bullshit, or they have to shut down their business because the landlord raised the rent and they can't afford it. **It's very rare that money brings you joy,** which makes me wonder if money really is the root of all evil? Nope, I don't think so! But the love of money is. It's what comes from money, the joy of taking care of people, paying your bills, providing, that makes the sacrifices worth it. I need and want money, not because I love money but I because I love the advantages and privileges that comes from having money. So yes, loving money may be destructive, but the love of what money can do will drive you to go that extra mile. Just make sure that mile is not leading you in the wrong direction.

Think of all you ever hear about money and money making, yet the money is rarely ever enough. You never hear people say, "I have enough money." They always want more. It's the way society has molded us as humans; we live life continuously having to make money, whether it be for personal pleasure, rent, food, clothes, transportation—it all costs money. Money brings opportunity, for instance, better schooling—not your average public school education. Money gives you a chance to live in a better neighborhood to raise your family. Shit, it costs money to die. Do you have $10,000.00 for a funeral put away or $2,000.00 for a decent headstone? Money can change your family for generations to come, if you make the right decisions with your money! I

"A wise person should have money in their head, but not in their heart." – Jonathan Swift

It's Not A Game

To get in the financial game, it is mandatory to set saving as a goal. Try to reach your goal a year from when you begin your Financial bag journey. Set what you feel is a realistic goal, but don't sell yourself short. Throughout the year, I set what I call 'Game Goals.'

In a basketball game there are 4 quarters, fouls, and mandatory TV timeouts. Apply the same rules to your yearly saving goal. The four quarters become a check in on your progress every three months. During these quarters are your timeouts. This is when you'll alter your spending. You'll be able to see where you went wrong, what you bought that wasn't a necessity, what you could've cooked at home instead of buying at a restaurant. Did you really need that purse? Did you really save from that Victoria Secret sale? Did you really need the Gucci flip flops? Also, in those timeouts, you figure out tactics for the rest of the game to fix the fuck ups. Halftime is a full break, revise your stats (credit score, remaining balance, bank account savings). In games, you have technical fouls. In this instance, a technical foul is a few things: blowing your whole refund/tax return on material things that have no resale value, excessively buying drugs and alcohol, having two girlfriends/boyfriends you have to provide for or spend on, celebrating holidays you don't believe in. At the end of the game (whatever date you set for your goal to be reached), you can only do one of two things: win or lose. If you tie, that's still a loss. The objective of a game in any sport is to score one more point than the opponent, and in this case the opponent is you. Fight temptation and save. You'll feel great when you see your credit score go up and your remaining balances go down.

"You know you must be doing something right if old people like you." – Dave Chappelle

Act Your Wage

Buy what you can afford, and go where you can afford. Stick to this rule whether you're buying clothes, going on a date, doing anything that isn't a necessity. The rule, "Don't buy one if you can't afford to buy two" relates to this. Stop spending money you don't have, while telling yourself the money you have coming in makes it okay to buy things you don't need. That isn't a winning formula, especially if the money you're dependent on is supposed to come from people paying you back what they owe. If you lend money, be prepared to lose that money. We know people aren't reliable, and everybody always wants to tell you about their hardships when they owe you money. Also, if you're waiting on payday every week, that isn't conducive to moving forward. You aren't saving, so you're living check-to-check.

The Financial bag will eventually guide you to having enough money and credit to own your own things. Whether it be your own car, house, or business, there's nothing like having your own. The importance of having your own is immeasurable. A simple example would be the difference between being a manager and the owner.

The Importance and Responsibility of Being the Boss

Know the difference between being a boss and being an over-seer. When you are the boss, you are responsible for all the fuck ups, not just your fuck ups. You are going to lose money, and have to figure out how to get it back. Overstand that you have to spend money to make money. When you were a worker or em-ployee, you might have been "fronted" or assisted. You're able to clock out when shift change comes, but when you own, there is no shift change. There is no day off. So, make sure the people around you respect your business and have your best interest or else you'll be fucked. Limit mixing friendship with business as much as you can. But on the other side of all the negative what ifs, it's the glory and pride of owning your own and being able to provide and build something from nothing.

Try not to mix your personal life with your financial life. Make sure your circle is filled with competitive people, but MAKE SURE they're actually competitive and not grimey. Make sure you're not associating with people who want to block each other from accomplishments but rather people who want to push one another to achieve things. Pushing each other to achieve things can come in many forms, minor bets or shit talking, whatever it takes for you to bust your ass. Michael Jordan improved not only because he worked out but because he also had great defensive teammates in practice. They were still on the same team, but they pushed each other to get better every day. You need that in your inner circle, that competitive motivation. I remember selling candy in elementary school. My best friend and I would always sell the most because I would come to school every day and say, "Ain't no way you selling more than me."

"I hate when niggas talk down on the trap, but they want every-thing that amounts from the trap."
– Kadeem Jackson

Enough for You Ain't Enough for Them

In high school, I went to school every day with snacks for sale. Not a small amount of snacks either. I'm talking about two igloo sized lunch bags filled with juice and sodas, two shopping bags and a backpack filled with chips, candy, and condoms. Yeah, condoms. For the whole year, I went to school without books in my bag, just things to sell. The senior class president, and the teacher in charge of the senior class complained to the principal about me messing up their business of selling snacks to raise money for prom. They told people not to buy from me. In spite of that, there I was every lunch wave and in between classes posted up with my snacks. Every day I made about $75 to $90 in profit. No one told me to save or explained the importance of it. So, I blew it all. Every weekend. For my high school readers or readers with family members in high school, tell them, "Get yourself a variety pack of candy from the wholesale spot or from Walmart, and do your thing, but make sure you save some of the profit."

This snack thing reminded me of two things regarding the Financial bag and Personal bag: know your friends, and pay attention to your money.

Shared Experience: For about a week, I noticed three of my friends, who would help me bring snacks to school, were nowhere to be found before or during school. When we would hang out after school there was an awkward energy I could feel. I didn't really say much because I didn't know what the vibe really was. As the days went by, I noticed I was leaving school with less snacks sold, but I saw more people with snacks. So, I went to the store and purchased a different brand of juice. The next day when I saw people with drinks I wasn't selling, I asked a friend who she got it from, but she didn't want to tell me. So, I asked someone who wasn't a friend of mine or theirs, and they told me who sold it them. She even told me when she bought it, the person selling it said, "Don't tell Splash you got it from me." Later that day, I noticed they all got on the bus but didn't get off on my stop, so I went to one of their house when they were all together, went to the fridge, and seen all juices that were being sold in school inside of the fridge. Their reason was I wasn't putting them on to make money, so instead they decided to do it themselves. No one really took the blame initially; they all blamed one another. I was confused because when I would go to the mall on the weekend, I'd buy them stuff too. They were my boys, so for simply bringing a bag into school so security would not turn me back, I'd purchase them a video game, a hat, a t-shirt, just about anything.

This was the first time I overstood that I can't make a person loyal just because I'm loyal to them. There are no rules to making money. Just because I have personal values, rules, and morals. That shit don't apply to anyone but me. In regards to the bozos, I just revamped my business by adding sodas, pop-tarts, and Pringles. Their business lasted about two more weeks, whereas mine lasted the whole school year because, for me, I respected the business and the hustle. They just wanted the money.

- Be able to acknowledge that there is a problem.
- Once the problem is identified, figure out how to fix the problem.
- Come up with more than one plan to give yourself a realistic chance at fixing the issue.
- Follow through with a plan.
- Find out where you went wrong and how this problem

could have been prevented.
- Make changes to avoid this problem from occurring again.
- Lastly, never blame the person. Take accountability for not seeing the issue sooner.

Keep your investment ideas to yourself. Don't end up being the guy who's pissed that you shared your idea with someone, and now they're putting it in motion. That's your fault. Protect your investment ideas. Your thoughts can all be monetary, but they can't just stay thoughts. Put them in motion. You have to figure out how you're going to present your product. Hit the drawing board, literally. Go to the store, and buy a whiteboard with a dry-erase marker and plot.

Everything we use on a daily basis was once just an idea. But everything is just an idea someone put into motion. That's how we now have cars, shoes, stores, pencils, chairs—all the simplest and most unique things we have. There's a saying, "The richest place in the world is the graveyard." It's true because all those people died with their plans and dreams that could have changed their families for generations—and possibly even changed the world. But that's not important. Worry about your craft. Master that.

"Empty pockets never held anyone back.
Only empty heads and empty hearts can do that."
– Norman Vincent Peale

Bag Challenge

- At the end of the day save everything in your pocket that's under a $10 dollar bill, coins included.
- Save $100 dollars on top of that every Friday or whatever set amount you can afford to consistently put aside. If you only walk around with your debit card, transfer your funds from your checking to your saving account at least $5 a day or just $100 each week.

If you want to intensify your saving routine for 30 days, follow the steps below:

- Don't go out for a month to a club, bar, movie, restaurant, mall, etc.
- Don't purchase any new clothing, footwear, or accessories if isn't for a job or opportunity to make more money.
- Every time you're invited to either of the above places or tempted to purchase something new, take that money and add it to your savings. For example, if you know you were going to buy the newly released Jordan or Yeezy shoes, add the total cost of the shoes to your savings.
- Finally, what I did to intensify my own saving tactic was, every time I was around someone who smoked, bought a drink, or anything unnecessary, I added what they spent to the savings. I did this to show to myself that if I tried to keep up with my surroundings, it would cost me X amount of dollars.
- At the end of the month, check what you saved and add that up. Multiply it by 12 and that is a rough assessment of how much you could save for the year.

The reason for this is to show you what trying to keep up with your friends will do if you are not financially careful and aware of your spending, especially because you are just doing things

130

to be down. There's nothing wrong with staying in your lane and missing out on a night or two out with friends. You have to keep your eyes on your bigger prize.

*"All I did was take my time, figure out where
I made a lot of mistakes and tried
not to make them no more."*
– Corey Woods

The Topsy Turvy Down Tree

When you have a goal or plan, you must have steps to complete your goal. Similar to having routes to your destination. You have to know where you want to go and how to get there, as well as when you'd like to be there. I like to think more of where I want to go than how I'm going to get there. I plan backward from the end goal to my current location. If the end goal is $100,000, I put the $100,000 at the top of the list and from there plan backward to how I'll get there.

A better way to think of it is like this: if you have a $100,000-dollar tree. The $100,000 is the root. The tree branches are the routes to your $100,000 dollars. All these investments, buying, selling, trading, and business risks are the branches. When you're done with that tree graph, look at the tree from an upside down perspective. Now that you're looking at it upside down, all those branches are the actions you must take to make it back to the root. Let me give you an example: if the end goal is to make $100,000 in one year, you have to make $8,333.33 a month. In order to make $8,333.33 a month, you have make to make $2,083 a week. You have to make $297.61 a day to make $2,083.33 a week. Start with the end goal, and dissect it. Know that everything is made up of parts that come together to make it whole. Know what bag you're trying to capture and the process of getting in the bag. Backward planning works with any goal.

"I'm from where your hustle determines your salary."
– William Leonard Roberts II

Ways To Fuck Up The Bag

1. Counting money you haven't yet made.
2. Buying one when you can't afford two.
3. Not knowing how to say NO when people want to borrow money.
4. Eating out instead of buying groceries.
5. Having too many credit cards.
6. Trying to keep up with people.
7. Quick-Flip schemes.
8. Ignoring the government; they will take your whole tax return.
9. Spending too much on a date with someone who isn't your partner and doesn't have a chance to be.
10. Buying something just because it's on sale.

*"Live in the lead, but work hard like
you're trying to catch up." – Robert Williams*

Imma Hustla

__*Splashism*__: Saving money is extremely important, but before you can save, you have to make money. **How can you save what you don't have? It's like securing something you haven't yet captured.** Knowing how to get money is the most essential component, there's a million things people want to invest in, own, build, and experience. The only problem is they don't have the funds. So, in order to pursue everything you want, you have to be able to generate money no matter where you are in life. Again, money should never define you. In the financial race, your monetary value and potential determines your monetary worth. How well you can monetize something determines your substance. Some people are natural born hustlers, some are survival hustlers, and some are learned hustlers. Which are you?

The Natural Born Hustler: The kid who sold everything even when they didn't realize they were selling something. If you are the natural born hustler, the clothes on your back are for sale, if someone offered enough. However, the natural born hustler struggles to turn the income into something because often, they never learned how to flip it into an investment.

The Survival Hustler: Their purpose isn't to get rich; it's to get by. Sometimes the Survival Hustler does too much at once and becomes a jack of all trades but a master of none. They do not mind, as long as they have a roof over their head and food to eat. A lot of you have this hustler in you, especially those of you coming from poverty. You know the feeling of not having anything, so, at any chance to have something, you jump at the opportunity.

This often leaves you in a situation where you are probably never financially stable enough to be set for life.

The Learned Hustler: This person is usually the most successful because they are taught from someone who has once been in their shoes and succeeded. The learned hustler knows who to learn from, and he surrounds himself with people wiser than him. Having been taught the common mistakes to avoid is what makes the him most privileged among the three hustlers.

"HOW CAN YOU SAVE WHAT YOU DON'T HAVE? IT'S LIKE SECURING SOMETHING YOU HAVEN'T YET CAPTURED."

"I've identified myself as a hustler since I was a young kid."
– Ermias Asghedom

Nipsey Hussle

Splashism: Nipsey Hussle encourages and endorses the notion of being your own boss, hence his slogan 'All Money In, No Money Out.' He got out of the deal and took his catalogue with him. For as long as I've been following Nipsey since 2008, everything about how he conducts himself has been the mannerisms of a BOSS. Although Nipsey isn't a mainstream artist or a household name yet, Nipsey is a boss. He is the head of his label 'All Money In,' and all decisions go through him. There is no asking for permission. He owns a clothing line and a store which is based in Crenshaw, which is where he is from. He owns a hair store in the same plaza. He also has his own strand of marijuana named "Marathon OG." In 2013, his street album 'Crenshaw' released on all mixtape platforms for free. He chose to charge $100 for a hardcopy of the tape. He launched a pop-up shop in his store for the album. The same album that would be free online sold about 1000 physical copies-in less than 24 hours. Before you close the book, look up Nipsey Hussle to see if I'm bluffing. Let me say that his next 'street album' made more history. He followed up 'Crenshaw' with 'Mailbox Money,' which he sold for $1,000. Yes, $1,000. He sold at least 60 copies a month before the same exact body of work was released for free. So, just imagine making $60,000 off a product people can receive for free. That's what bosses do—they get hands on and make you believe in the quality of their work. I'm pretty sure by the time you read this chapter, Nipsey will be a household name.

Similar to Nipsey Hussle, you should aspire to be the owner of something. If you're in the entertainment world, be the owner of your label. If you're into fashion, own your own brand, If you're into cooking, start your own cooking company. When you own your own, you don't have to make apologies to the media if you don't want to. You own you. You don't have to work with someone if you don't want to. You don't have to do anything you don't want to because your boss says so. That's the advantage of being like Nipsey. Everyone can't handle being the boss, but like Dame Dash says, "I can't respect people who bust their ass every day for a company for years—blood, sweat and tears—then has to get permission to go on vacation."[9] Nipsey is now part of a label, but as a partner to the label. He also spoke in an interview about how there were very good offers on the table, but he didn't take them because they would have only benefited him and not the partners who were with him from the start. Not jumping on an opportunity because it'll leave out people who were with you from jump is honorable! Since Nipsey is honorable and a boss who believes in his craft, he waited. He didn't sit on his ass. He put in work and built value, equity, and relevance while staying true to what was preached. You can't be out here leading the people and false prophesying. From what I've seen through Nipsey, you have to mix in the Spiritual bag with the Financial bag, stick to your beliefs, confidence in self, and build your equity. It'll give your business/brand substance. When your product is authentic, it has substance. The more focus and planning behind every move, the further your reach. The further your reach, the more lives you can impact.

"HE PUT IN WORK AND BUILT VALUE, EQUITY, AND RELEVANCE WHILE STAYING TRUE TO WHAT WAS PREACHED."

---

9   (Dash 2015)

"Never thought that I'd end up here.
Praying that God Made my pain disappear."
– Dashorn Whitehead

The 5 Tools Of Nipsey Hussle

1. *"I get money every day of the week. I go hard, I don't sleep.* You don't grind, you don't eat. In this world, my nigga ain't shit free."[10] You have to carry yourself as a boss, but work harder than your employees. If you're the worker, work harder than the employer.

2. *"Really came up in the field. Get money, get life, or get killed. Now how the fuck it's gone feel. When we start touchin' them mills…bet you the hustla' prevails. Equity all in my deal."*[11] Money doesn›t rule the world, but obtaining it on your own gives equity and validates what you have been saying even before you were paid.

3. *"This all I'm tryna do, hustle and motivate…hustle the Hova way. That's why they follow me, huh? They think I know the way. Cause I took control of things, ballin' the solo way. And if you counter my trend, I make you my protégé."*[12] When you know your financial plans and goals, believe in them and don't break. Push harder than ever to achieve them.

4. *"Quote me on this, got a lot more to prove. 'Member I came in this bitch, fresh out the county with nothin' to lose."*[13] Overstand the audience and meet their needs while taking risks that's worth the reward.

5. "*Cause ain't no point in playin' defense, nigga. That's why I dove off the deep end, nigga, without a life jacket. Couple mill', tour the world, dawg, my life crackin.' Cook the books, bring it back, so it's no taxes. Royalties, publishing, plus I own masters. I'll be damned if I slave for some white crackers.*"[14]
Never ever refuse to be the difference maker or to take a different approach!

"YOU DON'T GRIND, YOU DON'T EAT. IN THIS WORLD, MY NIGGA AIN'T SHIT FREE."

10	(Hussle, Let's Talk $ 2008)
11	(Hussle, The Field 2016)
12	(Hussle, Hussle & Motivate 2018)
13	(Hussle, Hussle & Motivate 2018)
14	(Hussle, Dedication 2018)

"Mysteries all in the pudding, and what's obvious is you only get out whatever you put in."
— Rayquon Elliot

Generational Wealth

There's a misconception that you have to be rich or wealthy to have generational wealth. Generational wealth builds over time, that's why it's generational. It has nothing to do with you reaping the benefits but everything to do with what you put in place for the generations that come after. There are many different approaches to obtaining generational wealth. **First, you have to start by developing some type of discipline and educating yourself** on the numerous investment options available to you. It's not about how much you make, it's about how much you save.

This is my suggestion:

1. Get life insurance. Within the policy, make it mandatory that the only way that the beneficiary can have any of this money is if they invest half of it into their children's life insurance. Also, make it mandatory that this continues for every generation to come after you. The goals are to set your family up to be more than taken care of, to be able to avoid debt, and to have a chance to make a difference and capitalize on financial opportunities that present themselves.
2. Saving for your children from birth is another way. Whether it be a single or two-parent household, saving $25 - $50 for your child from birth to age 18 gives your child a chance to start in the world of ownership at a young age, especially for children who don't want to go to college but have a passion in business.

3. Position yourself to be able to take advantage of investment opportunities: starting your own business, investing in an already established business, stocks and bonds, commercial and residential real estate, Roth IRA, just to name a few.

"Ask Steve Jobs wealth don't buy health."
– Terrence Thornton

Being Wealthy vs. Being Rich

The difference between being wealthy and being rich is simply this: rich people have one stream of income, and wealthy people have multiple streams of income. Wealthy people's money usually makes money for them while they sleep. Wealthy people tend to live within their means. You know, not as many purchased diamonds and jewels. Not as many exotic cars. Not as many flashy moments. Choosing to look wealthy over actually obtaining wealth is why a lot of people often end up being broke. It is essential that you find a way for your money to make money.

You have to find your inner hustler, which will unlock the enTRAPreneur tool. An entrepreneur is a person who organizes and operates a business or businesses, taking on greater than normal financial risks in order to do so. Do you know what it means to be trapping? Do you have a trap? Trapping is anything you need to do to make money. It could be selling cars, candy, or water on a hot summer day. Being a barber or a hairstylist is trapping. Being a personal trainer, promoting your product on Instagram, selling food in the summer are all trapping. If you're making money, you're trapping. The trap or trap house is wherever this trapping takes place.

Although the word originated from the streets and the drug dealing community, trapping doesn't mean you have to sell drugs. However, I'd prefer my family and friends to sell drugs, their body, or strip before being in the house without anything to eat or being able to even keep a roof over their heads. Whether your money is legally or illegally made, what you do with that money determines whether you are an enTRAPreneur or just trapping.

Look at the most successful people you know. I bet they don't work a 9-to-5. You have to be a go-getter. Wake up earlier. Maximize the 24 hours in a day when capturing and securing your bags. Remember what you had to sacrifice and change to reach your level of success to help you make the right decision within that split second of any temptation that could jeopardize it all! Not bashing anyone with a job. Just do that job well—shit, more than well! Be the DJ Khaled of selling cars. Be P. Diddy of your craft. When nobody is watching, whatever it is be one of the best to do the job.

"FIRST, YOU HAVE TO START BY DEVELOPING SOME TYPE OF DISCIPLINE AND EDUCATING YOURSELF."

"You define your own life. Don't let other people write your script." – Oprah Winfrey

Do What You Want When It's Yours

If you're working for someone and you feel like you're being underpaid, overworked, or unappreciated to the point you feel the bigger picture doesn't have you in it, LEAVE! Start your own business or go where you can get paid what you desire. Invest in yourself. Bet on yourself. Believe in yourself. Know yourself. Be yourself. I'm talking about investing with more than just money. You have to believe in the product (you). You have overstand the risk and be willing to take the risk. There's often a disconnect between the work people actually put in and their expectations. The work you put in is the hustle. This ain't about any get rich quick schemes, hitting the jackpot, or any of that fast money. It's about knowing your product inside and out.

You have to invest time and hustle into yourself and your financial plans. Then you need to act on it. Are you a person who tries or does? Are you going to leave your house on a hot summer day and sell 100 bottles of water or do you give up after a bad day? Are you going to study and find out which area needs your service the most, then go out and sell the water in those locations? Taking action is where you'll gain the trust of your consumers and yourself. No matter the task, after you sit down and brainstorm the genius ideas, brainstorm the execution and the possible gains and losses that can occur through the process of execution. The execution is what separates the doers from the tryers. Don't rush. Give yourself a higher success rate by being organized and prepared. Life is about a gamble. You know the saying, 'scared money don't make none'? Well dumb money don't make none either.

Don't ever let anyone guilt trip you out of making a better living for yourself. If you're taking time out of your day to do something and you can be making money off it, then do so.

"If you're a hater, we make you scared to show your face. It's called success." – William Leonard Roberts II

College

Splashism: I just want to say one thing: FUCK COLLEGE! Before you go to college or go back to college to finish up or to get another degree, decide if you really need this degree to do what it is you want to do. People are getting hired with no college degrees at places like Apple and Microsoft, and there's no ceiling on their income. Granted, you have to have a certain skill for these jobs, but it doesn't have to be a skill you obtained at a university. Overstand that debt collectors don't care if you can find a job with your degree or if you wished you studied something different because you do not want a job in that field anymore. As of the 2017 statistics, "Americans owe over $1.4 trillion in student loan debt, spread out among roughly 44 million borrowers. That's about $620 billion more than the total U.S. credit card debt. In fact, the average class of 2016 graduate has $37,172 in student loan debt, which is up six percent from last year."[15] An average of 37K means you could owe that for a job you have no real interest in or that is only available in an area you don't even want to relocate to.

I remember sitting, listening to all those college graduates with their bachelors, masters, and doctoral degrees—people talk about how much money they make, how great their job is, and how grateful they are to have a college degree. Never did I hear them talk about the debt you obtain while earning your degree. I see them in their late 40s early 50s or even later in life, finally getting their 'dream car' and finally doing what they want to do. You know, "The good ol' American Dream." Fuck that, we want to ball now, while we're young enough to enjoy it. Yes, I am a college graduate. Yes, I have debt. No, I didn't learn much in college that I feel benefited me in life. I went into college expecting and wanting to learn shit that would change my life for the present and the future. Look man, life is short, and I'm not saying college is the worst decision you can make, but you don't

---

15   (Student Loan Debt Statistics for 2017 2018)

need college to be successful. The system around us suckers us into basically believe seeing a UFO seems to be more realistic than succeeding without a college degree. So, they advertise college as if there is no other way to have success. I advocate for trades and hustles. Imagine life if you were taught actual entrepreneurial classes and budgeting in school, in addition to the trades you learned. Imagine having access to coding classes, home ownership classes, or something that would have been beneficial to your development.

Lastly, when the money's gone or when more rolls in, you'll still be you. The people around you will still be there. The universe will continue to rotate. Don't get a couple dollars and lose yourself. If you didn't take anything from the Financial bag, I hope you at least are wise and responsible enough to save your money for whatever life obstacles you come across, enough to give your kids everything you want. I pray, that as a member of this 5 Bag culture, opportunities for financial endeavors continuously fall into your lap, and you crush every chance to add generational wealth. As the great Kadeem Jackson once said, "The more they keep printing, the more we're going to make."

"My father told me 'Name your price in the beginning. If it ever gets more expensive than the price you name, get out of there.'" – Dave Chappelle

Financial Bag Questions:

1. How much money do you need to save until you reach your goal?
2. What new saving tactics are you going to use?
3. Can you handle the amount of money you hope for every day?
4. If you invest into one new thing what will it be?
5. Are you satisfied with your current bank account balance and credit debt?

_____
_____
_____
_____
_____
_____
_____
_____
_____
_____
_____
_____
_____
_____
_____
_____
_____
_____
_____

*"My biggest weakness is my sensitivity.
I am too sensitive a person."*
– Mike Tyson

This book is all about seeing and believing. Whether you know it or not, you control how you see yourself because your eyes don't see, you see with your eyes.

When you sit down, you see the seat and then you turn your back to the seat and sit. You no longer see the seat but you believed what you last saw, so you sit down freely. In retrospect, you believe what it is that your eyes see enough to sit without looking. So, when you look in the mirror, believe what you see, and if you correctly used the tools no one should be able to tell you that you are something you did not see when you last saw your reflection. You are forever able to adjust your mirror. These tools will always be in your possession.

Just because you have reached the end of this book it does not mean you have completely captured, secured, and fully gotten into your bag. If you've really paid attention to this book, every bag reminded you that actually being in your bag is a lifelong journey. So, instead of traveling on this journey alone, this book should be suggested to friends and family whom you notice are also not maximizing their full potential. The sooner you suggest this to them, the sooner they will be able to elevate, thus reuniting and vibrating on a higher frequency level with you. With that being said, this book should remain in arms reach and is definitely something you may need to refer back to when you notice that you have steered off your course. These tools will not work unless you do. You have to believe what you see when this mirror is built or no one else will. It is pivotal that you surround yourself with people who can be instrumental and have no issue holding you accountable.

My aspiration is that you are able to capture, secure, and get in your Spiritual, Mental, Personal, Health, and Financial Bag. Good luck on your bag journey. At any time, feel free to reach out to me or anyone who is a part of the bag culture!

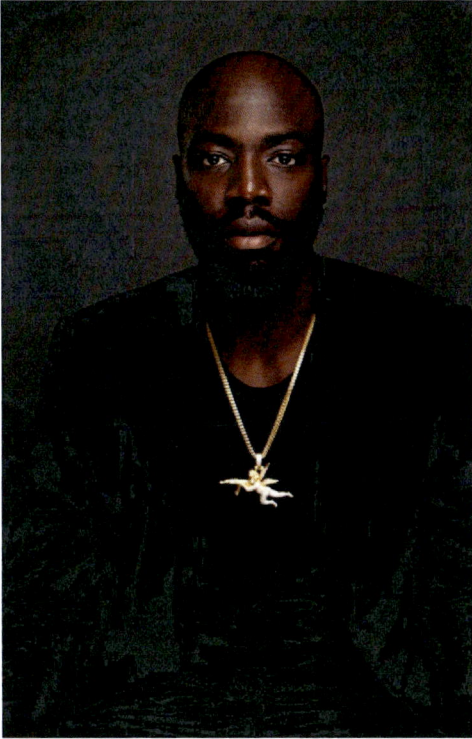

ABOUT THE AUTHOR

Maurice 'Splash' Eastwood educated at both Central Connecticut State University and the Streets of Hartford CT, where he is from—by way of Banbury, Jamaica (BAP! Bap!). He is a college graduate with a Bachelor of Art degree in Criminology, which he chose only to become an immigration officer to figure ways to get his family into the country faster. He is an inductee of 100 Men of Color, the first ever recipient of Firefighter Kevin L. Bell Heroic Award, a speaker, coach, moderator, a lover of basketball, yoga, therapy, meditation, dominos, music, pretzels, water, and everything debatable. He is an active staple in his community. He is a philanthropist, an enTRAPreneur, a community leader, a person who prides himself on genuineness, love, loyalty, honor, faith, and standing up for what you believe in. Maurice (Splash) also accepts money donations on his birthday (November 5th), which he always uses to buy toys for kids whose parents are deceased or incarcerated. Lastly, he organizes an Annual Back to School Supply Giveaway and is the coordinator of a Thanksgiving event, both servicing over 500 families.

Maurice (Splash) is reachable on
Instagram at MEastwood860
and Twitter at Meastwood860
also by email: Mauriceeastwood@gmail.com.

Books That I Recommend You Read:

How to Hustle and Win Part 1 by Supreme Understanding

How to Hustle and Win Part 2 by Supreme Understanding

Knowledge of Self by Supreme Understanding

Black God by Supreme Understanding

The Courage to be Disliked by Fumitake Koga and Ichiro Kishimi

The Lies My Teacher Told Me by James W. Loewen

The Millionaire Next Door by Thomas J Stanley

Fuck Feelings by Michael Bennet and Sarah Bennett

Get Your Sh*t Together by Sarah Knight

The Hustler's Ten Commandments by Hotep

Shook Ones by Charlamagne The God

The Misadventures of Awkward Black Girl by Issa Rae

The Outliers by Malcolm Gladwell

The Art Of War by Sun TZU

Dodging Energy Vampires by Northrup M.D., Christiane

Becoming by Michelle Obama

The Willie Lynch Letter and The Making of A Slave (PDF file available online for free)

Think and Grow Rich by Ben Holden-Crowther and Napoleon Hill

Unfu*k Yourself by Gary John Bishop

Contagious by Jonah Berger

Power vs. Force by David R. Hawkins